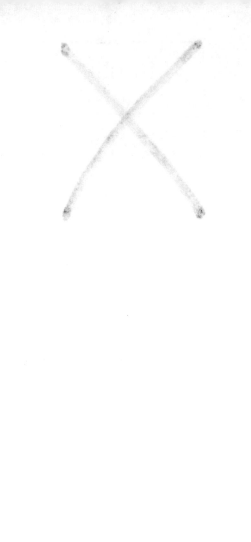

The
Leisure Literature

The
Leisure Literature
A Guide to Sources
in Leisure Studies, Fitness, Sports,
and Travel

NANCY L. HERRON
Editor

Contributing Authors
Adele F. Bane
Nancy L. Herron
Mila C. Su
Diane Zabel

1992
LIBRARIES UNLIMITED, INC.
Englewood, Colorado

Dedicated to the four families
who inspire and support us.

LIBRARIES UNLIMITED, INC.
P.O. Box 6633
Englewood, CO 80155-6633

Library of Congress Cataloging-in-Publication Data

The Leisure literature : a guide to sources in leisure studies,
    fitness, sports, and travel / Nancy L. Herron, editor ; contributing
    authors, Adele F. Bane ... [et al.].
        x, 181 p. 17x25 cm.
        Includes indexes.
        ISBN 1-56308-062-1
        1. Leisure--Bibliography. 2. Physical fitness--Bibliography.
    3. Sports--Bibliography. 4. Tourist trade--Bibliography.
    5. Travel--Bibliography. I. Herron, Nancy L., 1942-   . II. Bane,
    Adele F.
    Z7511.L37   1992
    [GV174]
    016.790'01'35--dc20   92-15144
                                                              CIP

CONTENTS

PREFACE

But the Gods, taking pity on Mankind, born to work, laid down the succession of recurring Feasts to restore them from their fatigue, and gave them the Muses, and Apollo their leader, and Dionysus, as Companions to their Feasts, so that nourishing themselves in festive companionship with the Gods, they should again stand upright and erect.

Plato

We have lived not in proportion to the number of years we have spent on this earth, but in proportion to the number we have enjoyed.

Henry David Thoreau

This book endeavors to identify, describe, and organize into a usable format 283 reference sources that support research related to leisure. The authors' major objective is to create a useful guide to resources that provides current information about leisure studies and data related to the three largest, fastest-growing leisure-related activities: sport, fitness, and travel/tourism.

In the last few years, international economic indicators have shown that worldwide spending on leisure-time activities contributed significantly to the growth of most national economies and that research activities related to leisure continued to increase steadily. But in spite of increased economic activity, heightened media exposure, and a proliferation of publications relating to leisure, no guide to that body of literature has emerged from the professional sector.

To fill that void, this working text was designed to familiarize researchers, students, faculty, librarians, and leisure studies professionals working in areas of leisure studies, sport, fitness, and travel/tourism with English-language resources available in today's information marketplace. This guide has been prepared by practicing subject specialist/reference librarians for fast and easy access to selected leisure resources, the best and most-used by professional information providers in all types of library environments.

In addition, this work has been designed as a teaching text for students wanting a clear, straightforward resource for learning about reference sources in each of these leisure fields.

Subject-specific annotated citations are grouped into four chapters, each consisting of two separate sections: (1) a treatise on the discipline, including a description of its reference environment and any unique aspects of its literature and (2) a fully annotated listing of some of the best, most-used titles arranged from the general to the specific in the areas of general leisure studies resources, sport resources, fitness resources, and travel and tourism resources.

In addition to print monographic and serial sources, descriptive annotated citations are also provided for microform, video, film, software, and online information resources. Each citation is provided with an alphanumeric code identifier for easy access to needed information; these in turn relate to the author/title and subject indexes following the text.

In the introduction to *The Social Sciences: A Cross-Disciplinary Guide to Selected Sources* (Englewood, CO: Libraries Unlimited, 1989), I spoke of discovering "new social science literatures growing out of the changes wrought from advanced computer technologies and the intense lifestyles of current populations." The literature of leisure has been identified as one of these. Neither clearly defined nor traditionally accepted as a separate field among the literatures of the social sciences, it is to date an amorphous mass of information in need of definition, organization, accessibility, and a sense of legitimacy. This book attempts to look at the literature of leisure as a newly emerging social science discipline—specific and unique unto itself—and to provide for that body of literature a first step toward legitimacy in the world of academe.

THE LITERATURE
OF LEISURE

Nancy L. Herron

INTRODUCTION

The concept of leisure has been present in established philosophical thought for centuries. Its value to mankind was well documented by the Greeks, and both Plato and Aristotle held the view that the proper use of leisure is one of the most serious of human concerns.[1] Friedrich Nietzsche,[2] Josef Pieper,[3] George Santayana,[4] John Dewey,[5] Lin Yutang,[6] Harry Allen Overstreet,[7] and Will Durant[8] all discuss the concept of leisure and its value to human existence. At the other extreme, leisure was a hotly debated topic among puritanical American thinkers of the early nineteenth century, many of whom were relatively isolated from cultural developments abroad. In their view, labor, whether necessary or not, was considered a virtue of patriotic Americans, whereas leisure was deemed a vice.[9] During the same period, in the more liberal-thinking environments of the British Empire, writers and thinkers often extolled the concept of leisure time. As early as the seventeenth century, Englishman Izaek Walton praised leisure-time activities extensively in his classic work *The Compleat Angler* (1653).[10] In the twentieth century, East Indian thinkers Shiyali Ramamrita Ranganathan[11] and Humanyun Kabir[12] came to look upon leisure as "a creative use of surplus time."[13]

Although the histories of Britain, Western Europe, and the East have for centuries demonstrated the historical presence of a leisure class, in America its rise was a relatively recent phenomenon, coinciding directly with the development of a rapidly growing prosperity and an improved awareness of technology as a result of the inventions of the Gilded Age.[14] The first major display of technological advances in the New World was the Centennial Exposition held in Philadelphia in 1876; it was at this international fair that Americans saw for the first time such modern-day wonders as the typewriter, Bell's telephone, Edison's multiplex telegraph, and the powerful Corliss Steam Engine.[15] Neither America nor American perceptions of work and leisure time would ever be the same; the United States had overnight become a modern nation.

Although the Exposition of 1876 began the process, the Columbian Exposition, held in Chicago in 1893, continued it. Considered by many to be the greatest achievement in America to that date, it had a powerful and far-reaching impact on the world's perception of America as an artistic and technological power and set the tone for present perceptions of leisure, its activities, and its place in lifestyles of the twentieth century and beyond.[16] Science and technology had, for the first time in human history, created conditions where human resources could cope with, if not outrun, human needs. New social standards were adopted by a rapidly growing urban population dominated by a group of prosperous individuals: the leisure class. Unlike their ancestors, who had condemned idleness, this social class valued leisure as a respectable sign of success. Thorstein Veblen, in his major sociological study *The Theory of the Leisure Class* (1899), described and analyzed this emerging class and established a means of categorizing and explaining its behavior.[17] Ronald Pisano, in *Idle Hours: Americans at Leisure 1865-1914*, capsulized Veblen's thought: Leisure was the "chief mark of gentility."[18] Stuart Chase, in the foreword to the 1961 edition of Veblen's work, stated that the purpose of Veblen's inquiry was "to discuss the place and value of the leisure class as an economic factor in modern life."[19]

The British historical perspective on leisure was presented in Stephen G. Jones's *Workers at Play: A Social and Economic History of Leisure 1918-1939*, which emphasizes the emergence of industrial capitalism, which imposed a number of new constraints on leisure—in particular, regular and longer working hours and new codes of organized and regulated recreation. These elements, Jones says, relate to wider themes of modernization throughout society.[20]

Following that theme, in 1980 Joffre Dumazedier, president and founder of the Committee on Leisure Research, International Sociological Association, spoke about the 1960s and 1970s from a leisure perspective. He believed that the leisure society of those decades rested on three specific social characteristics of that period:[21]

1. A steady increase in productivity enabled populations to pursue the paradox of industrial society: to produce ever more while working ever less.

2. A steady growth in the population's buying power made possible a great increase in leisure spending of the same magnitude as the growth in health care expenditures (accounting for income differences between the social classes).

3. An enthusiastic anti-technology movement had created a counter-culture centering around leisure time: a culture oriented no longer toward the standard of living but toward the style of living.

Dumazedier expanded the idea further to note that during the 1970s and 1980s new conditions developed that altered these characteristics:[22]

1. The rate of productivity tended to slow down and, at times, even decline. The energy crisis that first developed in 1973 offered little cause for optimism in the short run.

2. The consumption level tended to stagnate and unemployment increased.

3. The counterculture was no longer supported by a movement as homogeneous and dynamic as it was during the days of the beatniks and the hippies. It tended to be co-opted by the very system from which it sought to escape.

History has shown that the perception of leisure has changed over the past century, and predictions for the future have been repeatedly modified. But, according to Dumazedier, Thomas Kando's arguments against the hedonistic projections of Daniel Bell[23] and Herman Kahn[24] are the most compelling:

> One may only expect a moderate growth of time freed from occupational work by the year 2000. However, nothing indicates at the present time that the growth in leisure behavior and leisure values will come to a halt. It is true that in post-industrial economies where the services take up a majority of the labor force (over 50% in the United States and Canada), productivity grows more slowly. It is also true that the problems of leisure will differ, depending on whether the economy remains production-oriented and wasteful of natural resources or instead slows down production so as to give way to an orientation more respectful of nature and culture.[25]

Because we live in a transitional period, one dominated by McLuhanesque "global village" concepts,[26] solutions to more personal social problems, specifically those related to leisure concepts, tend to regularly elude governmental and policy decision makers around the world. An agenda that includes attention to special populations (the disabled, the aged, the educationally or socially deprived); depleted natural resources; environmental pollution; equal rights ideologies; the widening spectrum of acceptable lifestyles; and the increasing need for education for total living in an accelerated, technologically sophisticated world will be demanding attention in the twenty-first century.[27]

LEISURE'S TIE TO THE SOCIAL SCIENCES

The concept of leisure is found widely throughout the literature of the social sciences and has antecedents in all disciplines. Anthropologists, geographers, historians, philosophers, economists, sociologists, political scientists, and psychologists all have applied their discipline's research methodologies and vocabularies to the task of defining *leisure*. Sociologists have contributed the widest range of work on leisure. Their definitions of it have grown from a conceptualization of leisure as a solitary pursuit by an individual to the nature and role of free time activities by groups. Other academics, too, began to examine the role of leisure in molding an individual's identity, in working relationships, and in interpersonal relationships that develop among people functioning within a social unit—whether it be the family, the community, or the nation.

Most current definitions for leisure have been affected by the definer's perception of free time and how that time, free of work, is spent. In this text, leisure, as it is manifest in its literature, is defined by the authors as any activity accomplished during nonworking hours that has been chosen in relative freedom for its qualities of satisfaction for the individual. More specifically, leisure as similarly defined by John Kelly, is a "learned behavior, and is a central element in being human";[28] he believes that leisure is not peripheral or separate from the rest of life's meanings and relationships. He states that the leisure concept must be "crucial to our personal and social development and to our concepts of ourselves and the world about us. Its form and content transmitted in social context is a part of our culture, much more than just games and activities."[29]

Through time budget surveys conducted in the United States, Cuba, France, and the Soviet Union, we know that at least 90 percent of the time freed from occupational and household work is spent on leisure activities of all sorts at all levels, not including sociopolitical and socioreligious activities.[30] Leisure, then, is as leisure does.

LEISURE EDUCATION/ACADEMIC PROGRAMS

In 1868 Harry Barnard, the first U.S. Commissioner of Education, called for a form of leisure education in his *Biennial Report of the United States Commission on Education*: "The science of education includes the science of RECREATION and elaborate arrangements for the education of the community must be regarded not only as incomplete but radically unsound in which suitable provisions for physical training and recreation are not included."[31] Other important contributions to leisure education were made by John Dewey,[32] Charles D. Burns,[33] Anna May Jones,[34] Charles Brightbill,[35] Jean Mundy and Linda Odum,[36] and Norma J. Stumbo and Steven R. Thompson.[37] Stephen L. J. Smith[38] discussed broadening the view of leisure education to include the concept of leisure counseling. Arlin Epperson, Peter Witt, and Gerald Hitzhusen,[39] Larry C. Loesch and Paul Wheeler,[40] and E. Thomas Dowd[41] all contributed conceptual thoughts, principles, and applications to the practice of leisure counseling.

In 1934, Earnest E. Calkins published the *Care and Feeding of Hobby Horses*,[42] the first American bibliography of leisure activities, hobbies, and play. It was quickly followed in 1935 by Frederick J. Schmidt's *Leisure Time Bibliography: A Guide to Books and Magazine Articles Pertaining to Leisure Time and to Avocational Interests Related to Industrial Arts Education*.[43] In the late 1960s and 1970s, bibliographies of leisure literature began regularly appearing in support of formal classroom instruction in leisure studies at major research institutions in the United States, the United Kingdom, and Europe. This growing body of literature, much cross-disciplinary in nature, helped to claim legitimacy for leisure studies in traditional academe. Outstanding contributions were made by Marilyn Grace Guillaume, who produced her annotated bibliography of bibliographies on leisure in 1967,[44] and by Linda Lee Odum, with her 1977 annotated bibliography on leisure education.[45] The European Centre for Leisure and Education began its bibliographic series in Prague, Czechoslovakia, in 1970.[46]

Specialized journals related to leisure studies also began to appear, produced by organizations and academic institutions that had begun leisure studies departments in traditional colleges within the university structure. The first journal with a leisure concentration was a British one, *Leisure Manager* (formerly *LAM Journal* and *LAM*), produced by the Institute of Leisure and Amnesty Management, Cambridge, England, in 1936. By 1969, two more journals had emerged, *Society and Leisure: The Bulletin for Sociology*, a publication of the European Centre for Leisure and Education, and the American National Recreation and Parks Association quarterly, the *Journal of Leisure Research*.

The 1970s added several important titles: *Leisure Information Quarterly*, produced at the New York University Department of Recreation and Leisure Studies, premiered in 1972; in 1976 two British publications, *Leisure Futures*, a publication of the Henley Centre for Forecasting, and *Leisure Trade News* appeared. The American *Leisure Sciences: An Interdisciplinary Journal* followed in 1977 as did the Canadian quarterly, *Journal of Leisurability*.

A plethora of new leisure journals has appeared since 1980. *Leisure Lines*, a publication of the California Parks and Recreation Society, was first, in 1980; in 1981, *Leisure and Living*, a popular British magazine, and *Leisure Industry Digest*, the executive summary of current news in the leisure and discretionary spending markets, was published in Washington, DC; *Leisure Studies*, the organ of the British Leisure Studies Association, appeared in 1982, and *Leisure Intelligence*, a publication of the British Mintel Corporation, was born in 1983.

Within the last decade, extensive online databases of leisure studies information have been generated by both the public and the private sectors; this new approach to information access also attests to the legitimacy of the body of literature that is now called "The Leisure Literature." Most databases are available through vendor services: in the United States, DIALOG Information Services and BRS; and in the United Kingdom and Europe, CISTI, DIMDI, and the European Space Agency.

REFERENCE ENVIRONMENT

Today, the literature of leisure emphasizes current works but is not limited exclusively to them. Leisure concepts, like the theoretical basis of most disciplines within the social sciences, tend to build upon established cornerstones laid down by the important thinkers of past academic movements. It is upon this body of established thought that contemporary theory is being built.

Currently, leisure activities are being examined in new contexts. For example, leisure's commercial origins provide for the broadening of future national and international commercial enterprise. And mass media growth and technological innovation provide powerful mechanisms for increased control and manipulation of the industry. An excellent example of a publication that provides current perceptions of leisure is *For Fun and Profit*, a publication in which editor Richard Butsch brings together a series of contributed articles that link leisure to theories of consumption and commercialization.[47]

Like Butsch's work, the resources included in this text have antecedents in the literatures of ethics, trade, and the social sciences (geography, anthropology, economics, business, psychology, sociology, political science, law, and recreation); there are also ties to the fine arts, medicine, and technology. Although publications about leisure, sport, fitness, and travel/tourism are produced in all countries of the world and in all languages, the focus of this work is English-language resources, primarily those developed in the United States, Canada, and the United Kingdom, the three largest producers of leisure information in the world marketplace.

SOURCES

Guides and Handbooks

A-1.   Edginton, Christopher R., David M. Compton, and Carole J. Hanson. **Recreation and Leisure Programming: A Guide for the Professional**. Philadelphia, PA: Saunders College, 1980.

This guide was developed to reaffirm the importance of programming as the core element in the recreation and leisure service organization. It provides programming concepts, a discussion of the leadership role, the elements of planning, and suggested activities designed for success in recreational activities.

A-2.   Graefe, Alan, and Stan Parker. **Recreation and Leisure: An Introductory Handbook**. State College, PA: Venture Publishing, 1987.

In their handbook, Graefe and Parker have filled a need among leisure scholars, researches, and practitioners for a concise and useful information guide. The source is divided into two major parts based on geographic perspective: the first part deals with North American (United States and Canada) contributions to leisure studies, and the second part presents international perspectives. Especially important and useful are the descriptions of the disciplinary approaches, delivery processes, activities, environments, and population groups associated with leisure. An appendix of magazine and journal titles is provided.

A-3.   Jones, Anna May. **Leisure Education**. New York: Harper, 1946.

This dated but important classic was the first handbook created to help educators plan leisure education programs for the New York City schools. This work was viewed as a precursor of the contemporary leisure education movement and served as a model for future leisure studies texts, especially those dealing with leisure as a formal part of city school curricula.

A-4. Kimeldorf, Martin. **Pathways to Leisure**. Bloomington, IL: Meridian Educational Corp., 1989.

Kimeldorf designed his workbook to identify and suggest leisure activities and opportunities for free-time recreation.

Standard/Classic Sources

To begin this large category of important standard/classic sources, several highly acclaimed textbooks that explore elements of the study of leisure and leisure services head the list. These examples provide conventional and unconventional views of leisure and culture and of leisure and popular culture. Contributors present methodologies of time budget analysis and present survey measurement devices; they discuss holy days, holidays, and celebrations; they explore the life cycle, with emphasis on human behavior as it relates to leisure time; and they present the professional side of leisure and recreation.

A-5. Godbey, Geoffrey. **Leisure in Your Life: An Exploration**. 2d ed. State College, PA: Venture Publishing, 1985.

A-6. Godbey, Geoffrey. **Recreation, Park and Leisure Services**. Philadelphia, PA: Saunders College, 1978.

A-7. Godbey, Geoffrey, and Stanley Parker. **Leisure Studies and Services: An Overview**. Philadelphia, PA: Saunders College, 1976.

A-8. Sessoms, H. Douglas. **Leisure Services**. 6th ed. Englewood Cliffs, NJ: Prentice-Hall, 1984.

Selected standard and classic contributions include the following:

A-9. Bullaro, John J., and Christopher R. Edginton. **Commercial Leisure Services: Managing for Profit, Service, and Personal Satisfaction**. New York: Macmillan, 1986.

These two authors designed their book to help persons interested in developing leisure industry business ventures acquire grounding in leisure concepts, practices, and philosophies and to learn sound business practices related to the conceptual, theoretical, and practical elements of marketing and managing human and financial resources. There are nine chapters, an appendix containing a helpful dictionary of "computerese," and a subject index.

A-10. Charlesworth, James C. **Leisure in America: Blessing or Curse?** Philadelphia, PA: American Academy of Political and Social Science, 1964.

The foreword to this text reveals that the monograph grew out of a conference held in Philadelphia in 1963 that considered the issue of leisure and its place in the future lives of Americans. The speakers examined philosophical definitions of leisure, provided a comprehensive plan for wise use, and discussed the proper implementation of the plan. From a historical perspective, the publication is valuable for its interesting predictions of leisure time for the future.

A-11. Deem, Rosemary. **All Work and No Play? A Study of Women and Leisure**. Philadelphia, PA: Open University Press, 1986.

Deem presents a wide-ranging analysis of women's leisure in Britain. She discusses the complex relations among leisure, class, age, and race as well as the wide range of women's leisure experiences that currently exist. She also attempts to show how these different experiences have a common background in the constraints placed on women's leisure by men's expectations and by patriarchal culture.

A-12. Dumazedier, Joffre. **Toward a Society of Leisure**. New York: Free Press, 1967.

This is a classic work that focused academic sociology into its current dominant position associated with positive experience: liberty, fulfillment, choice and growth. Dumazedier defines leisure as follows: "activity — apart from the obligations of work, family and society — to which the individual turns at will for either relaxation, diversion or broadening his knowledge and his spontaneous social participation, the free exercise of his creative capacity" (p. iv).

A-13. Gillespie, Glenn A., ed. **Leisure 2000: Scenarios for the Future**. Columbia, MO: University of Missouri, 1983.

Gillespie's collection of eleven readings examines the issue of leisure in the context of change. The contributors focus on topics of socioeconomics, technology, professional issues, recreation, and tourism. They try to identify future trends in leisure studies that will need to be addressed in the classroom environment in the next century.

A-14. Glyptis, Sue. **Leisure and Unemployment**. Philadelphia, PA: Open University Press, 1989.

This title explores the darker side of leisure. Leisure has long been associated with the good things of life, says the author. But changing demographics, structural changes within the economy, the rapid adoption of new labor-saving technologies, and the deflationary economic policies of governments have contributed to the unleashing of unemployment as a dominant social and economic issue throughout the Western world. In this work, Glyptis examines several timely issues: the changing relationship between leisure and work; leisure policy and the community; unemployment; leisure participation patterns and lifestyles; and leisure provisions for the unemployed.

A-15. Gunter, B. G., Jay Stanley, and Robert St. Clair. **Transitions to Leisure**. Lanham, MD: University Press of America, 1985.

Gunter, Stanley, and St. Clair's book of readings focuses on the writings of several important authors, including Max Kaplan, that support a need for closer examination of leisure time in a societal context. The writers have attempted to identify three trends in contemporary society that underscore this fact: The first is the changing nature of the work day, the work week, and the work year; second is the growing proportion of the population reaching retirement; and third is a trend toward growth in involuntary unemployment. Copious references and general index provide a virtual "Who's Who" of the leisure literature.

A-16. Iso-Ahola, Seppo E., ed. **Social Psychological Perspectives on Leisure and Recreation**. Springfield, IL: Charles C. Thomas, 1980.

In this collection of important readings by such leaders in the field as John R. Kelly and John Neulinger, Iso-Ahola provides a set of original manuscripts designed to explore leisure and recreation from a social psychological perspective. In the introduction the editor states that the major goal of the text was the creation of a book "to advance the understanding of leisure and recreation behavior and offer a viable alternative to the conventional approaches to leisure and recreation."

A-17. Iso-Ahola, Seppo E. **The Social Psychology of Leisure and Recreation**. Dubuque, IA: William C. Brown, 1980.

Written by a social scientist with a social psychology perspective on the subject of leisure and recreation, this book was designed for use by college and university students as well as recreation practitioners. Although Iso-Ahola's perspectives in this volume are not unique, the extent of the coverage and the depth of the analysis contributed greatly to future developments in leisure studies programs and curricula in the later 1980s.

A-18. Kaplan, Max. **Leisure in America: A Social Inquiry**. New York: Wiley, 1960.

Kaplan's standard work laid down the modern definition of leisure and its place within human experience. Kaplan included the concept of "psychological freedom" along with five other concepts, including playfulness and pleasure expectation as part of the leisure experience.

A-19. Kaplan, Max. **Leisure: Theory and Policy**. New York: Wiley, 1975.

With its broad mixture of data, charts, tables, propositions, and hypotheses, this work set the standard for defining leisure in the 1970s. For the first time the ultimate issue in studies of leisure was defined as "the renewed study of human values as they are affected by the new leisure, especially industrially oriented leisure" (p. xix). The author identifies the objective of leisure as assisting man in mastering time—that is, himself.

A-20. Kelly, John R. **Leisure Identities and Interactions**. London: Allen & Unwin, 1983.

With this book Kelly makes a major contribution to the interpretive modes of sociological and social-psychological theory. The first text in the Leisure and Recreation Studies Series, this book provides a fresh analysis of leisure activities. Kelly demonstrates the importance of leisure to human development and traces its significance in the human life cycle. He also focuses on the kinds of leisure that are both most common and most significant—face-to-face encounters, family interaction, and activities that are part of our daily routines.

A-21. **Leisure and Life-Style: A Comparative Analysis of Free Time**. Edited by Anna Olszewska and K. Roberts. London: Sage Publications, 1989.

This work, which belongs to the Sage Studies in International Sociology Series, deals with leisure, its social and economic aspects, and its cross-cultural implications. Highlighted in the readings are important considerations such as hours of work and life-style differences across cultures.

A-22. **Leisure and Urban Processes: Critical Studies of Leisure Policy in Western European Cities**. Edited by Peter Bramhan et al. New York: Routledge & Kegan Paul, 1989.

Bramhan's collection of readings focuses on urban leisure policy in six of the liberal democracies of Western Europe. There are three major sections: Leisure, Politics and the City; Urban Initiatives in Leisure and Sport; and Leisure and Socio-Spatial Structure. The book includes many useful tables and figures as well as a bibliography and index.

A-23.   **Leisure Research: Current Findings and the Future Challenge**. London: The Sports Council in affiliation with The Social Science Research Council and the Leisure Studies Association, 1982.

This report of a joint seminar held at Imperial College, London, 1981, provides access to numerous papers and reports, workshops and documents, that describe the state of the art of leisure research projects completed in the United Kingdom.

A-24.   MacNeil, Richard D., and Michael L. Teague. **Aging and Leisure: Vitality in Later Life**. Englewood Cliffs, NJ: Prentice-Hall, 1987.

MacNeil and Teague offer a look at aging and present a discussion of some crucial questions relating to ever-increasing life expectancy. They also explore the principles of working with older adults and the kinds of leisure or recreation programs and services that promote physical, social, and emotional health.

A-25.   Neal, Larry L., ed. **Leisure Today: Selected Readings**. Reston, VA: American Association for Leisure and Recreation, 1973.

This monograph reprints articles from the first eight issues of *Leisure Today*. The articles first appeared in the *Journal of Physical Education and Recreation* for the months of March and June, 1972; January, June, and November/December, 1973; April and November/December, 1974; and May, 1975. Themes include changing concepts of leisure, research and thought about children's play, leisure and the environment, urban concerns, creative programming, community education, the concept of lifestyles, and recreation for special populations.

A-26.   Neulinger, John. **The Psychology of Leisure**. Springfield, IL: Charles C. Thomas, 1981.

A revision of the 1970 first edition of this classic scholarly work on the psychology of leisure deals with such issues as the conceptualization of leisure, its measurement, research methodologies and findings, social indicators, attitudes, challenges, problems, and qualities. Numerous tables, appendices, bibliography, author and subject indexes complete this important work.

A-27.   Neulinger, John. **To Leisure: An Introduction**. State College, PA: Venture Publishing, 1984.

Neulinger's textbook is designed to introduce the concepts of leisure studies, that is, leisure education and leisure counseling, to readers exploring the subject for the first time. Two examples of leisure surveys are provided. Appendices and an extensive bibliography and index complete the volume.

A-28.   Neumeyer, Martin, and Esther S. Neumeyer. **Leisure and Recreation: A Study of Leisure and Recreation in Their Sociological Aspects**. New York: A. S. Barnes, 1949.

This important work provided an informed framework for the acceptance of recreation and leisure into modern society. It is a study of leisure and recreation's sociological aspects, but it is not limited exclusively to the sociological viewpoint. The authors provided a basis for leisure research and methodology that has been used by succeeding researchers in the field of leisure studies.

A-29.   Osgood, Nancy J., ed. **Life after Work: Retirement, Leisure, Recreation and the Elderly**. New York: Praeger, 1982.

Like other titles in this category, this monograph grew out of a conference. "Life after Work: Retirement, Leisure, and the Elderly" was held at the State University of New York at Cortland in 1981. The topic was chosen because of recent demographic changes and modifications in the nature of work; the institution of retirement; labor force participation rates; and changes in the political, economic, legal, and family structures in U.S. society.

A-30.   Parker, Stanley. **The Sociology of Leisure**. New York: International Publications Service, 1976.

This sociological inquiry into leisure extended the relationship between work and leisure roles. The book is divided into three parts, each representing different approaches to the subject of leisure: part 1 considers the context in which leisure has developed; part 2 consists of an examination of the relationship between leisure and other spheres of life; and part 3 deals with practical concerns, including areas in which sociology meets social administration planning and the more social concerns of such people as geographers and economists.

A-31.   Pieper, Josef. **Leisure: The Basis of Culture**. New York: New American Library, 1963.

At the end of World War II, Pieper wrote this classic work on the nature and role of culture in modern life (originally published in 1952). Often labeled an elitist view of leisure, it contends that leisure time is for contemplation, reflection, meditation, and/or joyous celebration. Contemporary recreational activities would not meet Pieper's standard of "true" leisure or culture.

A-32.   Pruette, Lorine. **Women and Leisure: A Study of Social Waste**. New York: Arno Press, 1972.

This monograph is a reprint of a 1924 study and a part of the series American Women: Images and Realities. It is noteworthy for the social and moral questions the author asks about women and leisure, about men's perceptions of women as being unfit for leisure activities, about women's role in the family, and about women's place in the world of work.

A-33.   Rojek, Chris, ed. **Leisure for Leisure: Critical Essays**. Basingstoke, England: Macmillan Press, 1989.

Rojek's collection of critical essays, in addition to being informative, points to new directions for discussion and research in leisure and leisure studies. Eleven contributing authors explore what the editor calls "the world beyond the conventional wisdom" of the traditional leisure literature.

A-34.   **Values and Leisure and Trends in Leisure Services**. State College, PA: Venture Publishing, 1983.

This collection of papers written by members of the Academy of Leisure Sciences is a testimony to scholarship in leisure studies. The nine topics included were selected for their value in advancing leisure education, for exploring societal trends that influence recreation and leisure, and for their contributions in documenting the values of recreation and leisure for the individual and society. The outstanding scholars in leisure studies can be counted among the Fellows of the Academy.

A-35. Wade, Michael G., ed. **Constraints on Leisure**. Springfield, IL: Charles C. Thomas, 1985.

In the foreword to this monograph, Michael Ellis of the University of Oregon states that this is one of the few modern books on leisure and its related phenomena that starts from the premise that leisure is a desired state of mind that accompanies voluntary behavior. He states later that the contributions to this book broadly adhere to the notion that leisure is a voluntary enterprise, whether that is expressed strictly through observable behavior or in a more experiential or abstract terms. The book falls into three parts: part 1 deals with the psychological constraints that impinge upon leisure; part 2 focuses on a socioeconomic perspective of leisure constraints; and part 3 builds on both the intra- and interpersonal factors that are discussed in the two previous parts, using these as a backdrop for an examination of the potential leisure-oriented constraints throughout the lifecycle.

A-36. Winnifrith, Tom, and Cyril Barrett. **The Philosophy of Leisure**. New York: St. Martin's, 1989.

Winnifrith and Barrett concern themselves with tracing the philosophical and aesthetic roots of the modern concept of leisure. They present papers that, for the most part, were presented at the Philosophy of Leisure Conference held at the University of Warwick in 1986.

Dissertations

A-37. **Dissertation Abstracts International**. Ann Arbor, MI: University Microfilms, 1938- . Online and CD-ROM formats available.

Approximately 35,000 doctoral dissertations from more than 500 institutions are indexed annually in this source. Accompanying abstracts are author-prepared. The index is published in three separate parts: "Section A: The Humanities and Social Sciences"; "Section B: The Sciences and Engineering"; and "Section C: Worldwide." Dissertations are organized under broad categories that are subdivided. Two indexes are provided: author and keyword. Unfortunately, the keyword indexing approach often requires users to search under many terms in order to find dissertations on a given topic. The online and CD-ROM formats are often preferable to the printed index, because they provide greater searching flexibility and are relatively easy to use. Most of the dissertations indexed in *Dissertation Abstracts International* may be purchased in print or microfilm format from University Microfilms International. (See entries B-19, C-18, and D-13.)

Bibliographies and Catalogs

Two early classic bibliographies on leisure time activities exist. Although dated, they have been included here because they set a standard and produced a model for what would follow in annotated bibliography:

A-38.   Calkins, Earnest E. **Care and Feeding of Hobby Horses**. New York: Leisure League of America, 1934.

A-39.   Schmidt, Frederick J. **Leisure Time Bibliography: A Guide to Books and Magazine Articles Pertaining to Leisure Time and to Avocational Interests Related to Industrial Arts Education**. Ames, IA: Iowa State College, 1935.

Important later contributions to bibliography include the following:

A-40.   Guillaume, Marilyn Grace. **An Annotated Bibliography of Bibliographies in English on Leisure, Recreation, Parks, and Related Topics and an Analysis of Bibliographic Control**. M.S. Thesis. Chicago: University of Illinois, 1967.

A-41.   Kaplan, Max. **Leisure, Recreation, Culture and Aging: An Annotated Bibliography**. Washington, DC: National Council on the Aging, 1982.
        This work has as its major purpose the assembling of the most significant works in the subject areas of leisure, recreation, culture, and aging. One hundred and sixteen entries on such topics as activities, theories, institutions, minorities/subcultures, programs, psychology/sociology, research findings, and demographic trends are presented. The final product confirms that the compiler was successful in setting the newest direction in gerontology and in aligning it with the humanities and arts.

A-42.   Odum, Linda Lee. **Annotated Bibliography on Leisure Education**. Arlington, VA: National Recreation and Parks Association, 1977.
        The emphasis of Odom's bibliography is on leisure education. It includes curriculum materials designed to advance leisure education projects.

A-43.   **Recreation and Leisure Data Files**. Machine Readable Archives. Canada: Public Archives, 1983.
        The Machine Readable Archives is one of eight divisions in the Archives Branch of the Public Archives, Canada, and is responsible for appraising, acquiring, and controlling computer files of historical/research value. Most of this file relates to recreation and leisure, and the data provided were generated from the results of surveys conducted by Parks Canada among the users and visitors to its national parks and historic sites. The printed format is in English with French text on inverted pages.

Dictionaries and Encyclopedias

A-44.   **Leisure, Recreation and Tourism Abstracts Word List**. Wallingford, United Kingdom: Commonwealth Agricultural Bureaux International, 1990.
        The LRTA word list is a register of the terms used in the subject index of *Leisure, Recreation and Tourism Abstracts* (entries A-55, C-47, and D-25) and the terms used in the descriptor field of the database of this British indexing and abstracting service. It has been compiled with two major objectives in mind: to assist the online and offline interrogator of LRTA and to constitute the basis for a hierarchically organized thesaurus of leisure and related terms.

A-45.   Smith, Stephen L. J. **Dictionary of Concepts in Recreation and Leisure Studies**.
New York: Greenwood Press, 1990.

Described by the author as a "verbal" map of the world of recreation and
leisure studies, this is the first comprehensive concept dictionary for the field. About
100 terms are grouped into four broad, overlapping categories: elemental concepts,
theoretical concepts, research or methodological concepts, and professional concepts.
Each term is defined and accompanied by an in-depth, chronologically arranged discussion linking it to others in the volume. Handy cross-referencing is provided and
numerous scholarly references are given for expanded research. This book is an
outstanding contribution and will be established as a standard in the field of leisure
studies.

A-46.   **Social Science Encyclopedia**. Edited by Adam Kuper and Jessica Kuper. New
York: Routledge & Kegan Paul, 1985.

The *Social Science Encyclopedia* covers many newer and more specialized
concepts that cannot be found in earlier, more comprehensive works like *International
Encyclopedia of the Social Sciences* (17 vols. New York: Macmillan, 1968) or *Encyclopedia of the Social Sciences* (15 vols. New York: Macmillan, 1930-35). Leisure subjects
and their antecedents can be traced here and much information is available in the 700
articles covering the fields of anthropology, economics, political science and political
theory, psychology, demography, development studies, linguistics, semiotics, and
psychiatry. Business and industrial relations, communication and media studies,
geography, medicine, and women's studies are also included. Articles were contributed
by 500 scholars from twenty-five countries, with many coming from the United States,
the United Kingdom, and Europe.

Directories

A-47.   **Directory of Canadian University Data Libraries/Archives**. Compiled by Anna
Bombak and Charles Humphrey. Edmonton, Canada: University of Alberta
Data Library, 1990.

The compilers state that the purpose of this directory is to provide information
on major Canadian academic centers of precollected machine-readable data, their
services, and collections. The directory is compiled from information submitted by
individual Canadian university-affiliated data libraries and archives. Directory entries
are arranged alphabetically by university name. A summary table of data library/
archive user services and a contact list of machine-readable data resource persons are
provided.

A-48.   Smith, Michael A. **Directory of Leisure Scholars and Research**. Salford, United
Kingdom: Centre for Leisure Studies, University of Salford, Annual.

This directory lists the approximately 500 members of the Centre for Leisure
Studies; membership is worldwide, although the largest number come from the United
Kingdom. Name and address, research interest, publications, and professional asso-
ciation membership are provided, as is an index of leisure interests.

Indexes, Abstracts, and Databases

A-49. **Academic Index**. Foster City, CA: Information Access Company, 1976- . Monthly Updates. Online and CD-ROM formats available.

    The *Academic Index* database provides indexing of more than 400 scholarly and general interest publications. It covers the most commonly held titles in college and university libraries and includes information on the areas of social sciences and the humanities. The subject coverage includes the following: art, anthropology, economics, education, ethnic studies, government, history, literature, political science, general science, psychology, religion, sociology, and leisure studies.

A-50. **Applied Social Sciences Index and Abstracts (ASSIA)**. London: Library Association, 1987- .

    The *ASSIA* is international in scope, covering more than 500 English language journals from sixteen countries, with more than 80 percent originating in the United States or the United Kingdom. Although the emphasis is on the traditional disciplines of the social sciences, frequent citations relating to leisure concepts, studies, and activities are included. The main body of the index consists of citations arranged by subject in a form of chain indexing (linked subject entries in which the full entry is found under the main topic and cross-references are made from the others). Each citation includes standard bibliographic information and an abstract of approximately 150 words.

A-51. **Cendata**. Washington, DC: U.S. Bureau of the Census. 1980- . Current, daily updates. Available online.

    Statistical data, press releases, and product information from the Bureau of the Census, U.S. Department of Commerce are provided in this important database. Subjects covered are often peripheral to leisure studies but can provide important hard-to-find statistical data. Subjects include agriculture, business, construction and housing, trade, governments (national and international), manufacturing, population, and much more. Demographic data include excerpts from *Current Population Reports*, the *1980 and 1990 Census*, and limited data on more than 200 countries.

A-52. **Current Index to Journals in Education (CIJE)**. Phoenix, AZ: Oryx, 1969- . Monthly, with cumulative annual index. Online and CD-ROM formats available.

    This abstracting service functions through the Educational Resources Information Center (ERIC), begun in 1964 by the federal government to serve as a clearinghouse for educational information. ERIC indexes educational journal articles and reports and maintains an extensive database of information that is available on paper or in electronic formats, including CD-ROM. Information relating to leisure topics is often found by using this source and its descriptors. (See entry B-37.)

A-53. **Education Index**. New York: H. W. Wilson, 1929/32- . Monthly, except July and August, with quarterly and annual cumulations. Online and CD-ROM formats available.

    The primary emphasis of this tool is subject and author indexing to more than 325 education periodicals, selected monographs, serials, and government publications.

It provides access to many citations in the leisure literature. This is a useful source of current information, because most articles included have been indexed within one to three months of publication. (See entry B-38.)

A-54. **Educational Resources Information Center (ERIC)**. Washington, DC: Affiliated with the U.S. Department of Education, Office of Educational Research and Improvement, 1966- . Monthly updates. Online and CD-ROM formats available.

ERIC is the complete database providing over 700,000 citations on educational materials from the Educational Resources Information Center. The database corresponds to two print indexes, *Resources in Education* (*RIE*) (entry A-58) and *Current Index to Journals in Education* (*CIJE*) (entry A-52). It can be used effectively to find information related to the research and pedagogical aspects of leisure studies. (See entry B-40.)

A-55. **Leisure, Recreation and Tourism Abstracts**. Wallingford, United Kingdom: Commonwealth Agricultural Bureaux, 1976- . Quarterly. Available online.

Although recreation and tourism citations seem more predominant, leisure is one of the major subject areas covered in this important British indexing and abstracting service. The scope of coverage is worldwide, providing access to citations in both English and non-English language journals. All abstracts are in English. This service is an important resource for leisure studies information found in such journals as *Journal of Leisure Research* (see entries A-63 and D-39), *Journal of Leisurability* (see entry A-62), *Leisure Management*, *Leisure Sciences* (see entries A-68 and D-41), *Leisure Studies* (see entry A-69), *Society and Leisure* (see entry A-71), and *World Leisure and Recreation* (see entries C-47 and D-25).

A-56. **PAIS International in Print**. New York: Public Affairs Information Service, 1991- . Monthly. Online and CD-ROM formats available.

PAIS International in Print replaces two important indexes used to locate information related to public affairs: *PAIS Bulletin* and *PAIS Foreign Language Index*. Subjects covered in this database include economics, law, political science, business, public administration, transportation, and international relations. Many of these subjects relate to leisure studies and this source can provide a wealth of information on leisure and leisure-related activities worldwide. Included are all types of materials, especially those dealing with governmental bodies, such as pamphlets, reports, and conference proceedings. Books and articles from more than 1,400 periodicals are regularly included. (See entry D-27.)

A-57. **Psychological Abstracts**. Princeton, NJ: American Psychological Association, 1927- . Online and CD-ROM formats available.

This publication, developed by the American Psychological Association, summarizes the world's serial literature in psychology and related disciplines such as anthropology, sociology, and communications. The electronic component, *PsycLIT*, expands the coverage of the bound version by including dissertations and non-English language entries. Much information relating to leisure studies and its research components can be found in this important resource.

A-58. **Resources in Education (RIE)**. Phoenix, AZ: Oryx, 1975- . Monthly, with annual and multi-year cumulations. Online and CD-ROM formats available.

Whereas *CIJE* (entry A-52) concentrates on journal articles, *RIE* covers other types of educational materials that support education and instruction. It is a good source of information on curriculum materials associated with leisure studies. Materials covered include unpublished and published research reports, papers presented at conferences, in-house documents, tests, questionnaires, and selected government publications. *RIE* is a product of the ERIC database.

A-59. **Social Sciences Citation Index (SSCI) / Social SciSearch.** Philadelphia, PA: Institute for Scientific Information, 1969- . Triannual. Online and CD-ROM formats available.

The *SSCI* is composed of three major components: *Permuterm Subject Index*, *Source Index*, and *Citation Index*; it is the *Citation Index* that enables a searcher to look for any publication (by author, then date and source title), regardless of publication date and format, and to learn whether other authors cited that publication in their work during the period covered by the *Citation Index*. The *Permuterm Subject Index* allows the searcher to look for items published in the year covered in the index under every significant word or phrase in the title paired with every other significant work or phrase in the title. The *Source Index* provides full citations to both citing articles listed in the other two indexes. The comprehensive and interdisciplinary nature of the indexes and their wide scope (1,400 social sciences journals and 3,100 additional journals) makes this an important tool for leisure studies researchers. In addition to paper format, this index is available online as "Social SciSearch" from 1972. An important feature in the electronic format is its ability to search the author's cited references in addition to the more conventional retrieval by title words, source authors, journal names, and corporate source.

A-60. **Sociological Abstracts.** San Diego, CA: Sociological Abstracts, Inc., 1953- . 5 issues/yr. Online and CD-ROM formats available.

This important resource is the premier index to the literature of sociology and indexes 1,600 journals in related disciplines. International in scope, it provides much information on published documents related to leisure and leisure studies. Coverage includes original research, reviews, discussions, monographic publications, panel discussions, and case studies. Conference papers and dissertations are also indexed. In the paper format two separate supplements index book reviews and conference papers. (See entry D-31.)

A-61. **Sociology of Education Abstracts.** Abingdon, England: Carfax, 1965- . Quarterly.

For those seeking leisure studies information with an international coverage, this source may be helpful. It covers approximately 300 journals, many of them British, and includes monographs and yearbooks within its scope. About 600 abstracts per year are produced with each running about 100 to 200 words in length.

Core Journals

A-62. **Journal of Leisurability**. Islington, Canada: Leisurability Publications, 1980- . Quarterly. Indexed in *Leisure, Recreation and Tourism Abstracts*.

Each issue of this quarterly Canadian journal has a distinctive title, but its main interest is with leisure and recreation as they apply to the handicapped. Special attention is given to leisure services, but economic issues and those appealing to facilities managers are often highlighted.

A-63. **Journal of Leisure Research**. Alexandria, VA: National Recreation and Park Association, 1968- . Quarterly. Indexed in *Leisure, Recreation and Tourism Abstracts*.

This major research organ, co-published by the University of North Texas, provides scholarly articles related to all facets of leisure and leisure education. (See entry D-39.)

A-64. **Leisure Futures**. London: Henley Centre for Forecasting, 1976- . Irregular.

The Henley Centre's publication appeals to the business and economics, banking and finance side of leisure studies. It provides economic data and statistical analysis of information generated from leisure trend indicators.

A-65. **Leisure Industry Report**. Washington, DC: Leisure Industry Recreation News, 1981- . Bimonthly.

Formerly titled *Leisure Industry Digest*, this publication is an executive summary of current news on the leisure and discretionary spending markets of the world.

A-66. **Leisure Information Quarterly**. New York: New York University, 1972- . Quarterly. Indexed in *Rural Recreation and Tourism Abstracts*, *World Agricultural Economics and Rural Sociology Abstracts*.

Formerly *Leisure Information Newsletter*, this publication is produced by the Department of Recreation and Leisure Studies.

A-67. **Leisure Manager**. Cambridge, England: Turner Associates, 1936- . Indexed in *Leisure, Recreation and Tourism Abstracts*, *Rural Recreation and Tourism Abstracts*, and *World Agricultural Economics and Rural Sociology Abstracts*.

One of the oldest serials dealing with leisure issues, this title is produced by the Institute of Leisure and Amenity Management, Cambridge, England, and articles presented cover all aspects of parks management. Circulation is about 4,000.

A-68. **Leisure Sciences: An Interdisciplinary Journal**. New York: Taylor & Francis, 1977- . Quarterly. Indexed in *Leisure, Recreation and Tourism Abstracts*, *PAIS International in Print*, *Communication Abstracts*, *Geographical Abstracts*, *Human Resources Abstracts*, *Sage Urban Studies Abstracts*, and *Rural Recreation and Tourism Abstracts*.

One of the most scholarly of the leisure journals, *Leisure Sciences* has an interdisciplinary approach. All aspects of leisure are covered in depth, but focus is mainly academic, with articles on the theoretical and conceptual aspects of leisure studies. (See entry D-41.)

A-69. **Leisure Studies**. London: E. Spon and F. N. Spon, 1982- . 3 issues/yr. Indexed in *Leisure, Recreation and Tourism Abstracts*.

This publication, a product of the British Leisure Studies Association, focuses on detailed aspects of leisure and provides a vehicle for ideas associated with academics, social issues, and topics that relate to the leisure policy and leisure studies curricula in Britain and Western Europe.

A-70. **LSA Newsletter**. Leeds, United Kingdom: Leisure Studies Association, 1980- .
Quarterly. Indexed in *Rural Recreation and Tourism Abstracts* and *World Agricultural Economics and Rural Sociology Abstracts*.

Formerly the *LSA Quarterly*, this product of the Leisure Studies Association, Leeds Polytechnic Unit, Carnegie School, has its focus primarily on academic perspectives on leisure issues.

A-71. **Society and Leisure**. Prague, Czechoslovakia: European Centre for Leisure and Education, 1969-76(?). Indexed in *Leisure, Recreation and Tourism Abstracts*.

The subtitle for this publication is *Bulletin for Sociology of Leisure, Education and Culture*. It was published by the European Centre for Leisure and Education in cooperation with the Committee for Leisure and Popular Culture of the International Sociological Association. It continues as *Loisir et Société / Society and Leisure* (Presses du l'Universite du Quebec, Canada, 1978-). This publication is a humanities and social sciences journal devoted to the academic study of leisure in various societies.

Conference Proceedings

A-72. The Academy of Leisure Sciences. **Annual Forum Proceedings**. State College, Pennsylvania, 1980- . Annual.

Although work was begun in 1973, the Academy did not come together as a unit until 1980 for the purpose of advancing the understanding of leisure through discussion, debate, and exchange of ideas. The interdisciplinary Academy carries out this purpose through an annual forum plus the reporting and publishing of research and scholarly papers devoted to exploration and critical analysis of leisure in a changing society. Members come from the fields of business, education, humanities, science, social science, and recreation and parks.

A-73. American Association for Leisure and Recreation (AALR). **Proceedings of the Annual Conference**. Reston, Virginia, 1974- . Annual.

This association was established by the American Alliance for Health, Physical Education, Recreation and Dance as a support for (1) college and university teachers of recreation and park administration, leisure studies, and recreation programming; (2) professional recreation and park practitioners; and (3) people involved in other areas of health, physical education, and recreation. Among its goals is nurturing the conceptualization of the philosophy of leisure through curriculum development and professional preparation. The association publishes a newsletter, *The AALR Reporter*, and two journals, *Journal of Physical Education, Recreation and Dance* (see entries B-51 and C-51), and *Leisure Today*.

A-74. Commission on Education of the World Leisure and Recreation Association (CEWLRA). **Proceedings of the Annual Conference**. Sharbot Lake, Canada, 1968- . Annual.

As a commission of the World Leisure and Recreation Association, this body seeks to educate people working in recreation and related fields. It publishes *World Leisure and Recreation*, quarterly; a semiannual newsletter; and a journal, *International Directory of Academic Institutions in Leisure, Recreation and Related Fields*, printed in English, French, German, and Spanish.

A-75.   Commission on Research of the World Leisure and Recreation Association (CRWLRA). **Proceedings of the Annual Conference**. Champaign, Illinois, 1978- . Periodic.

CRWLRA is composed of research and policy officers, universities, and government organizations for the purpose of supporting leisure research through conferences and exchange. It is affiliated with the World Leisure and Recreation Association, a parent organization.

A-76.   Leisure Studies Association (LSA). **Proceedings of the Annual Conference**. Leeds, United Kingdom, 1976- .

The association, established in Britain at Leeds Polytechnic Unit, Carnegie School, meets annually at various institutions of higher education throughout Britain. Included among past conference themes are the following: Forecasting Leisure Futures, Leisure and the Community, Leisure and Learning in the 1980s, and Leisure and the Media.

A-77.   National Recreation and Park Association (NRPA). **Proceedings of the Annual Conference**. Alexandria, Virginia, 1965- . Annual.

The association is a public interest organization dedicated to improving the human environment through improved park, recreation, and leisure opportunities. The themes of past conferences reflect these interests as well as topics stressing research, technical assistance programs, public policy, and leisure education. The association has an extensive publication program including four monthly and two quarterly journals, *Journal of Leisure Research* (see entries A-63 and D-39) and *Therapeutic Recreation*.

A-78.   World Leisure and Recreation Association (WLRA). **Proceedings of the Annual Conference**. Sharbot Lake, Canada, 1956- .

This organization is a multinational, international service agency that provides assistance to nations seeking to provide recreation service to their citizens. It maintains membership in fifty-three countries and acts as an information clearinghouse, conducts research, and holds conferences and symposia. Its publications include *International Directory of Academic Institutions in Leisure, Recreation and Related Fields* (periodic), *International Directory of Leisure Information Centers* (periodic), and *World Leisure and Recreation* (quarterly).

Statistical Sources

A-79.   **American Statistics Index**. Bethesda, MD: Congressional Information Service, 1973- . Monthly, with annual cumulations. Online and CD-ROM formats available.

This important publication providing citations to statistical information produced in publications of the U.S. Government is presented in two separate parts: one is an extensive index volume and the other volume contains abstracts for the citations. Statistical data on all aspects of leisure studies can be found in this source, which emphasizes demographic data of all types. (See entries C-77 and D-53.)

A-80.   **The Lifestyle Marketplanner**. Wilmette, IL: Standard Rate & Data Service, National Demographics & Lifestyles, 1988.

This statistical compilation joins demographic information for the top 100 areas of dominant influence (ADI) markets with data on fifty of the most popular lifestyle activities in the United States. It continues as *Lifestyle Market Analyst* and its data are assembled from the results of market survey findings.

A-81.   Watson, William G. **National Pastimes: The Economics of Canadian Leisure**. Vancouver, Canada: The Fraser Institute, 1988.

Watson's study examines the broadcasting, cable-TV, film, recording, and performing arts services associated with leisure time in Canada. It explores leisure issues associated with sector growth, with change, and with relative pricing effects of the industry. Part 1 examines the industries, their growth sectors, and relative pricing effects; part 2 addresses policy concerns. Appendix tables provide information on industries covered in the study, major expenditure aggregates, personal recreation expenditures, recreation expenditures by income group, price and wage data, employment and labor force data, and employment in various entertainment-related occupations.

NOTES

[1]Humanyun Kabir, "Foreword," *Leisure and Recreation in Society*, by Zulie Nakhooda (Allahabad, India: Kitab Mahal, 1961), i.

[2]Friedrich Wilhelm Nietzsche, *Nietzsche*, trans. Martin Heidegger (London: Routledge & Kegan Paul, 1981).

[3]Josef Pieper, *Leisure, the Basis of Culture* (New York: New American Library, 1963).

[4]George Santayana, *The Philosophy of George Santayana* (New York: Scribner's, 1953).

[5]John Dewey, *The Later Works, 1925-1953*, ed. Jo Ann Boydston (Carbondale, IL: Southern Illinois University Press, 1981).

[6]Lin Yutang, *Chinese Essays* (Seoul, Korea: Chinwadang, 1986).

[7]Harry Allen Overstreet, *A Guide to Civilized Leisure* (New York: W. W. Norton, 1934).

[8]Will Durant, *The Foundations of Civilization* (New York: Simon and Schuster, 1936).

[9]Ronald G. Pisano, *Idle Hours: Americans at Leisure 1865-1914* (New York: Little, Brown, 1988), 1.

[10]Izaek Walton, *The Compleat Angler* (New York: Heritage Press, 1948).

[11]Shiyali Ramamrita Ranganathan, *Education for Leisure* (London: Asia Publishing House, 1961).

[12]Kabir, i.

[13]Ibid., i.

[14]Pisano, 3.

[15]Ibid., 3.

[16]Ibid., 3.

[17]Thorstein Veblen, *The Theory of the Leisure Class* (New York: Modern Library, 1931).

[18]Pisano, 1.

[19]Stuart Chase, "Introduction," *The Theory of the Leisure Class*, by Thorstein Veblen (New York: Modern Library, 1961).

[20]Stephen G. Jones, *Workers at Play: A Social and Economic History of Leisure 1918-1939* (London: Routledge & Kegan Paul, 1986), 1.

[21]Joffre Dumazedier, "Foreword," *Leisure and Popular Culture in Transition*, by Thomas A. Kando (St. Louis, MO: C. V. Mosby, 1980), vii.

[22]Ibid., vii.

[23]Daniel Bell, *Toward the Year 2000: Work in Progress* (Cambridge, MA: Beacon Press, 1970).

[24]Herman Kahn, William Brown, and Leon Martel, *The Next 200 Years: A Scenario for America and the World* (New York: Morrow, 1976).

[25]Dumazedier, viii.

[26]Marshall McLuhan and Bruce R. Powers, *The Global Village: Transformations in World Life and Media in the 21st Century* (New York: Oxford University Press, 1989).

[27]Janet R. Maclean, James A. Peterson, and W. Donald Martin, *Recreation and Leisure: The Changing Scene* (New York: Macmillan, 1985), ix.

[28]John R. Kelly. *Leisure* (Englewood Cliffs, NJ: Prentice-Hall, 1982), v.

[29]Ibid., v.

[30]Dumazedier, vii.

[31]Steven L. J. Smith, *Dictionary of Concepts in Recreation and Leisure Studies* (New York: Greenwood Press, 1990), 188.

[32]John Dewey, *Democracy and Education* (New York: Macmillan, 1916).

[33]Charles D. Burns, *Leisure in the Modern World* (New York: Century, 1932).

[34]Anna May Jones, *Leisure Time Education* (New York: Harper, 1946).

[35]Charles K. Brightbill, *Educating for Leisure-Centered Living* (Harrisburg, PA: Stackpole, 1966).

[36]Jean Mundy and Linda Odum, *Leisure Education: Theory and Practice* (New York: Wiley, 1979).

[37]Norma J. Stumbo and Steven R. Thompson, eds., *Leisure Education, A Manual of Activities and Resources* (Peoria, IL: Central Illinois Center for Independent Living and the Easter Seal Leisure Resource Center, 1986).

[38]Smith, 189.

[39]Arlin Epperson, Peter Witt, and Gerald Hitzhusen, eds., *Leisure Counseling: An Aspect of Leisure Education* (Springfield, IL: Charles C. Thomas, 1977).

[40]Larry C. Loesch and Paul Wheeler, *Principles of Leisure Counseling* (Minneapolis, MN: Educational Media Corp., 1982).

[41]E. Thomas Dowd, ed., *Leisure Counseling: Concepts and Applications* (Springfield, IL: Charles C. Thomas, 1984).

[42]Earnest E. Calkins, *Care and Feeding of Hobby Horses* (New York: Leisure League of America, 1934).

[43]Frederick J. Schmidt, *Leisure Time Bibliography: A Guide to Books and Magazine Articles Pertaining to Leisure Time and to Avocational Interests Related to Industrial Arts Education* (Dubuque, IA: Iowa State College, 1935).

[44]Marilynn Grace Guillaume, *An Annotated Bibliography of Bibliographies in English on Leisure, Recreation, Parks and Related Topics and an Analysis of Bibliographic Control* (M.S. Thesis, University of Illinois, 1967).

[45]Linda Lee Odum, *Annotated Bibliography on Leisure Education* (Arlington, VA: National Recreation and Park Association, 1977).

[46]European Centre for Leisure and Education, Bibliographic Series (Prague, Czechoslovakia: The Centre, 1970).

[47]Richard Butsch, *For Fun and Profit* (Philadelphia, PA: Temple University Press, 1990).

THE LITERATURE
OF FITNESS

Adele F. Bane

INTRODUCTION

Fitness has meant many things over the years.[1] Even today, there is no universally accepted definition of *fitness* in the context of *health-related* physical fitness.[2] Contemporary definitions of fitness in terms of exercise and health depart from the earlier and more traditional concept of fitness as *motor fitness* or "physical abilities that relate primarily to athletic performance."[3] A typical definition of health-related physical fitness describes it as a state characterized by: "(1) an ability to perform daily activities with vigor, and (2) traits and capacities that are associated with low risk of premature development of the hypokinetic diseases (i.e., those associated with physical inactivity.)"[4]

It is also difficult to define fitness because related terms are often used interchangeably with it. For example, *health* and *fitness* have almost become synonymous in everyday usage.[5] Health in this sense is considered a "human condition with physical, social, and psychological dimensions."[6] *Fitness* and *wellness* also tend to be used synonymously in corporate settings where wellness is "a holistic concept" describing an individual's positive state of health deriving from biological and psychological well-being.[7] The wellness concept borrows from perspectives of the 1960s to construct a view of fitness that takes into account the condition of the mind, body, and spirit. It is here especially that we see the multidimensional nature of health-related fitness.

The definition of fitness has evolved with the movement. The current fitness boom began in the 1970s and stabilized in the 1980s. The beginnings of the 1970s movement are not unanimously attributed to any particular series of events. One source, the *Facts on File Dictionary of Fitness*, attributes the "genesis" of the movement to the 1972 Olympics, when Frank Shorter, an unknown American runner, won the gold medal in the marathon. This event was believed to inspire thousands of ordinary people "to jog on the highways and byways" in search of the rewards of staying fit.[8]

Another scenario suggests that during the late 1960s and early 1970s, Americans were disillusioned with medical science and realized that medicine could not be relied upon to prevent death—especially from heart disease. There was also dissatisfaction with the "social disintegration" of the time and tension created by the Vietnam War and civil rights issues. Social scientists suggest that the jogging craze became a way to exorcise the deficiencies of the time and that fitness was heralded as a way to protect individuals from the characteristic ills of a turbulent era that fostered stress, substance abuse, and depression.

Momentum for the fitness movement grew in the mid-1970s when Dr. Kenneth Cooper discovered *aerobics*, the system of exercise that involves vigorous movement and the goal of increasing oxygen consumption. Cooper's book, *Aerobics*, details his scientifically developed program of exercise.[9] The potential health benefits of physical fitness were further etched into the public's awareness by Jim Fixx's book, *The Complete Book of Running: A Layman's Approach to Long Distance Running.*[10]

By the end of the 1970s, medical research confirmed the positive effects of exercise on health and hinted at the possibility of increased longevity as well. These research results fueled the revolution, and today pollsters estimate that 75 million Americans exercise on a regular basis.[11]

In the 1980s, the running/jogging movement matured, and exercisers learned that aerobics should not be the only consideration in a fitness regimen. This was graphically illustrated by the untimely death of author Fixx while jogging. Obviously, aerobic conditioning could not provide all the most important fitness benefits alone. Experts advised that it should be accompanied by other elements such as nutritious diet, stress control, and risk management.[12]

An emphasis on health-related physical fitness came with the 1980s. Aimed at physical education teachers, the *AAHPERD Health Related Physical Fitness Manual* included a definition of the concept that now focused on health-related components instead of on functional capacity without mentioning the exercise/health linkage. The President's Council on Physical Fitness and Sports also expanded its definition of physical fitness to include a healthy lifestyle. Being physically fit was defined as "the ability to carry out daily tasks with vigor and alertness, without undue fatigue, and with ample energy to enjoy leisure time pursuits and to meet unforeseen emergencies."[13] Educators stressed that all fitness experiences should be designed to promote a positive attitude toward fitness. The attitude component gained importance as studies continued to indicate that fitness was related to self-confidence, self-esteem, and self-discipline.[14]

In tandem with the American people's personal interest in fitness, and spurred on by the rising costs of medical care, corporations began to pay renewed attention to the health of their employees and the economic benefits of fitness programs. Wellness programs were developed to link physical fitness with health promotion. Health promotion activities were a combination of health education and related organizational, economic, and environmental supports designed to achieve behavior conducive to well-being.[15]

Modern corporate wellness programs had their roots in earlier physical fitness programs started at the turn of the century. In the 1880s, John R. Patterson, president of National Cash Register, regularly assembled his employees at dawn for prework horseback rides. In 1941, the National Employee Services and Recreation Association (NESRA) was formed. It encouraged employee recreation programs to enhance employee health. NESRA estimates that by the late 1980s more than 50,000 organizations had some type of physical fitness program with about 300 employing full-time fitness directors.[16]

During the 1950s, sports and recreation had been the focus of organization-sponsored wellness programs. By the 1970s, formalized physical fitness programs and corporate athletic facilities began to appear. These early workplace wellness programs concentrated on health conditions that could be influenced by modifying behavior: smoking, weight reduction, cholesterol reduction, high blood pressure control, and exercise habits.

By the late 1970s and early 1980s, a broader definition of fitness was incorporated into the employee health movement. Suddenly, concepts like "individual responsibility, corporate wellness culture and holistic (mental, spiritual and physical) health, also fit under the umbrella of wellness."[17] Health was no longer just an absence of disease. Experts in the 1980s looked at health from a much broader perspective. Health would be measured in terms of degrees on "the wellness continuum."[18] Those at the positive end of the continuum would have good health and the ability to enjoy life while those at the negative end would be experiencing ill health and, in the extreme, mortality.[19]

Most wellness programs included at least one of these forms of intervention: education, medical screening, prescription programs, and behavior modification support services such as equipment and classes. Because wellness programs were preventive in orientation, they differed from more traditional employee assistance programs that offered treatment for problems such as substance abuse.

Fitness in the 1990s will focus on empowerment. "Health power" will move out of the doctor's office into the home, school, and office.[20] As evidenced by spending patterns, new health habits are a part of the American lifestyle. In 1988, Americans spent approximately $77 billion on diet foods and vitamins alone. Consistently, exercise videos are among the top ten selling home videos, and magazines such as *American Health*, *Prevention*, and *Self* each report circulations in excess of 1 million.[21]

Authorities writing in the field suggest that the twenty-first century definition of fitness will focus on self-directed awareness and action aimed toward integrating physical, emotional, social, and spiritual life to achieve optimal performance within our environment.

RELATED AREAS OF STUDY

The body of fitness knowledge, concepts, and skills is borrowed from a variety of disciplines, including health education, physical education, human movement studies, sports, sociology, biochemistry, anthropology, leisure studies, and recreation. Authors who have written fitness books acknowledge assistance received from colleagues in the fields of exercise physiology, health promotion, medicine, psychology, and education. Fitness books and journals are often indexed under one of these related terms rather than having an independent fitness subject descriptor.

In the literature, a close relationship exists between physical fitness and sport because the health goals of sport are similar to those of fitness/wellness. They include building character, promoting better health, and bringing communities together.[22] Shared information resources are common — for example, the fitness bibliographies produced by the Sport Information Resource Centre (SIRC). The 1987 Sports Participation Survey by the National Sporting Goods Association (NSGA) can be used to profile typical fitness participants. The survey found that people with higher education levels tend to be more active in fitness activities, but higher income levels do not similarly influence participation.[23] And sporting goods sales are an indicator of the popularity of specific fitness activities.

A relationship also exists between medical science and exercise science. Occupational health professions often do medical screening for corporate wellness programs and are a good source for evaluation studies of these programs. Of course, these studies can "run the gamut from relatively simple reports of physiological responses of participants to full-blown cost-analyses that weigh the costs of program administration and implementation against the benefits in terms of dollars and sense."[24] For an example of the more in-depth type of study, see the Blue Cross and Blue Shield of Indiana *Health Promotion Service Evaluation and Impact Study*.[25]

Cardiologists involved with exercise physiology laboratories contribute persuasive research results on the link between health and fitness practices. Dr. James Rippe, working at the University of Massachusetts Medical Center, studied the fitness habits of 1,139 top executives to establish the correlation between fitness and maximum performance. This study became the basis for his book, *Dr. James M. Rippe's Fit for Success*.[26]

Epidemiologists have also contributed proof of the health benefits of exercise. In one study by Ralph S. Paffenbarger, Jr., 1,700 Harvard alumni were studied over a period of many years to assess the long-term health benefits of lifestyle elements of college students and alumni. In 1986, he reported that it is physical activity as an adult, not as a college athlete, that is associated with a reduced risk of death in Harvard alumni.[27] Another study led by Dr. Steven Blair of the Institute for Aerobics and the Cooper Clinic found that "even becoming modestly fit ... can dramatically reduce one's chances of dying from cancer, heart disease and other afflictions."[28]

School health classes touch often on fitness/wellness concerns, because the goal of health education is to provide "any combination of learning experiences designed to predispose, enable, and reinforce voluntary adaptations of behavior conducive to well being." And health education combines with health promotion "to influence environmental, organizational, and economic supports" for positive lifestyle behaviors.[29] The same goals apply to fitness education, and health educators are among the leading providers of fitness information at all levels of schooling.

Looking at fitness from a societal perspective, sociologists are often the most compelling in proving that fitness has moved from fad to mainstream. They ponder the sociocultural appeal of fitness practices, products, and ideology.[30] And sociologists, alone, caution about the possible downside of having corporations holding title to more of the employee's "selfhood" through corporate wellness programs, because these programs give the corporation new claims on the employee's body and at the same time the "space between work time and private time has narrowed."[31]

The related discipline of psychology has been brought to bear on fitness motivation and behavior. Programs offered to individuals or workers that promote psychological and emotional health are incorporating a behavioral component to encourage open communications, rational thought processes, and a positive outlook.[32]

Leisure and recreation trends are mentioned frequently in relation to fitness activity analyses. Marketers to the fitness industry analyzing the future of fitness centers must have knowledge about the resources and lifestyles of a particular market segment. When the Canadians recently studied fitness participation, they examined statistical data on travel, tourism, outdoor recreation and family expenditures, and supplemented those data with surveys of physical activity habits.[33] Generally, these areas are considered together when exploring issues related to the "managed recreation industry."[34]

FITNESS CONSUMERS

The fitness boom of the 1970s and its accompanying personal health craze stabilized in the 1980s and became mainstreamed in the 1990s. The value Americans place on fitness mirrors the value they place on their bodies and their self-image. The "me" generation is "frightfully fit" and considers health and well-being pressing matters.[35] The fit body "holds a signal position in contemporary American culture—as locus for billions of dollars of commercial exchange and a site for moral action."[36] The popularity of aerobics continues and fitness gurus regularly promote books, videos, and their own television programs. Autobiographical accounts by fitness celebrities in books and magazines bear witness to the power of fitness in overcoming life's problems (drug abuse, depression, and eating disorders). Everyone, at any age, is encouraged to take part in popular physical activities like swimming, tennis, walking, and cycling.[37]

Americans are persuaded that exercise will bring order, health, and accomplishment into their lives. Swimming, walking, and running/jogging have become the activities of choice. Fitness walking, stationary cycling, soft (nonimpact) aerobics, swimming, and treadmill exercise accounted for nearly 15 million new fitness participants in 1988.[38] Outdoor swimming has been popular since recreation surveys began in the 1960s. Swimming enthusiasts cite fitness benefits and socialization as their incentives. Pleasure walking was tied with swimming as the most widespread activity in the 1982-83 *Nationwide Recreation Survey* (NRS). As evidenced by the NRS and other surveys, the pervasiveness of running and jogging in American life can only be described as extraordinary.

Because the number of Americans over sixty steadily increases, elder fitness emerges as a growing market for the fitness industry. Even the youngest baby boomers are approaching forty and have started to see their own physical decline. Because the major illnesses today are not infectious but chronic and degenerative — and hence responsive to prevention and treatment by exercise and diet — boomers are leading the fitness revolution.[39]

Entire communities have benefited from the fitness incentive. Health awareness came to Wellsburg, West Virginia, in May, 1988 when the Bayer Company inaugurated its wellness program there. This health education campaign was designed to lower the risk of heart disease through behavior modification. By 1989, citizens of Wellsburg lost over two tons of weight, reduced their average cholesterol by almost 20 points, and 44 percent of smokers had quit. Bayer is developing a how-to guide for other interested communities.

Corporate culture has adopted wellness with a passion. The sheer bulk of journal literature attests to the popularity of this concept in corporate America. Issues that brought and keep worksite health promotion in the fore-front include the desire to keep valuable employees and reduce employee turn-over, rising health insurance costs, and lagging productivity. Corporate leaders also know that such programs enhance the organization's image among workers and in the community.[40]

Although the number of companies with health education continues to grow, specific programs vary greatly. Among America's most visible corporate wellness programs are:

1. Bonnie Bell, which began its first official fitness program in 1976. It offers a wooded jogging path, classes, tennis courts, and exercise facilities.

2. L. L. Bean, which believes in its health and fitness program enough to spend $200,000 per year on it. Managers cite productivity gains as the major benefit to the company.

3. AT&T, which currently has 80,000 employees who have volunteered for their Total Life Concept (TLC) program. Its motto: "A healthy workplace makes good business sense."

4. Sara Lee, where six companies based in Winston-Salem, North Carolina, center their wellness programming around women's health issues because 80 percent of their workforce is female. This focus is relatively new in wellness programming.[41]

Other major wellness program leaders are Control Data Corporation, PepsiCo, Kimberly-Clark Corporation, Johnson & Johnson, IBM, Xerox, Sentry Insurance, and Tenneco. The Tenneco program has won top ratings from the Washington Business Group on Health and the Association for Fitness in Business. Employees pay nothing for this program, which offers extensive physical facilities, thirty-two classes a week, fitness testing, and individual counseling on all subjects.

Johnson & Johnson's Live for Life program is designed to encourage employees to adopt lifestyles that result in good health. The program began in 1978 and the company spends $200 per employee annually on its headquarters fitness program. The company is so convinced that wellness programs will continue to be an important corporate strategy to contain health care costs that it opened a Health Management division to market the "Live for Life" program to other companies. Johnson & Johnson has become a leader in fitness consulting to corporations. Its biggest competitor is Execu-Fit Health Programs, begun in 1983 by Karen Behnke. Using her knowledge of fitness and health, Behnke designed a health promotion program for corporations. She compiled convincing data on how much unhealthy employees cost their employers. Clients took notice. Execu-Fit now has 125 clients in thirty states.[42]

There are a variety of approaches and resources available to companies that wish to provide some type of wellness program. Fitness consulting companies now design programs to fit any company's budget, facilities, and objectives. On-site screenings are provided by private firms that specialize in corporate health services. The medical component can be provided by occupational health professionals from area hospitals and clinics. Companies without fitness facilities often contract with a local fitness center for a corporate group discount. Companies often get interested in health when one key person—often the chief executive officer—gets enthusiastic. One CEO is tapping his own company's resources. Ralph Guild's company, Interep Radio Store, is the only corporation in New York with its own private dance studio, a staff director of dance, a live jazz pianist, and a chairman who takes an hour out of his day to tap with his employees—everyone from secretaries to executives.

Joseph Kotarba says there are some negatives to avoid in wellness programming. Employers should not offer the most prestigious, individualized, and costly preventive care services to their executives while offering group and classroom programs to their staffs. Companies should seek overall participation by employees, because it has been found that those most likely to participate are those whose "style of self" already recognizes the value of wellness activities.[43] On an average, programs attract under 20 percent of the work force. Exercise programs tend to be more popular among white collar workers while blue collar workers tend to have less healthy lifestyles. Critics say that programs are not reaching those who need them most.[44]

Evaluating the impact of a wellness program is plagued with problems of methodology.[45] Descriptive research can contribute "to basic knowledge about health beliefs, attitudes, values, and behavior, as well as to epidemiological knowledge of the distribution and etiology of disease. Similarly, good evaluation can contribute to the store of research knowledge about the fundamental relationships between specific interventions and specific changes in comprehension, motivation, behavior, and health outcomes in specific populations."[46] A model for a descriptive study is the Rippe survey of the fitness behavior of top executives, which used a questionnaire supplemented by selective interviews. As a model for a formal program evaluation, the Blue Cross and Blue Shield of Indiana (BCBSI) study of their health promotion service should be reviewed. Characterized by its designers as a "quasi-experimental design," it was "nevertheless able to quantify and measure many critical variables." At the same time, it serves as a "practical wellness model" that is easy to duplicate.[47]

For the most reliable cause and effect data, longitudinal studies that measure the same group of individuals at different times over a long period are preferred over the more popular and less time-consuming cross sectional design, which compares different groups of people at the same time.[48] Because the focus of current health research has shifted to "chronic and degenerative diseases ... current results require even more waiting and sensitive measurement."[49] This approach was taken in the College Alumni Study, a long-term follow-up of nearly 17,000 Harvard alumni over twenty-five years. The study, conducted by Dr. Ralph Paffenbarger and his colleagues, provided "solid evidence" that lifelong, consistent exercise provides important cardiac health benefits as well as enhancing daily life.[50] A more detailed discussion of research techniques in the health sciences can be found in these sources: *Measurement and Evaluation in Health Education and Health Promotion* by Lawrence W. Green and Frances M. Lewis and *Research Techniques for the Health Sciences* by Laurna Rubinson and James Neutens.

It is generally agreed that the most effective wellness programs have a dual focus. They provide information and skills to individuals and modify the workplace environment to encourage productivity and reduce stress.[51]

Looking ahead, fitness professionals envision continued growth for fitness programs in the 1990s. Whether in the home, fitness center, or workplace, an "amalgam" of programs, equipment, and services will be needed for a diversified, growing population of people who want to be fit for life.[52]

INFORMATION ENVIRONMENT

The subject of health and fitness has received scant attention in the literature until recent years.[53] There is an expressed need to "enlarge our understanding of this complex phenonmenon of which we continue to be a part."[54] It is only within the last three decades that physical conditioning and physical fitness have been given much attention by the American public. President John F. Kennedy has been given credit for spurring this awareness in the 1960s, and the President's Council on Physical Fitness and Sport continues to promote interest in the topic, especially among schoolchildren.[55]

In some critical areas of fitness research, the need for further study has been documented. For example, there are gaps in our knowledge about how young children respond and adapt to physical exercise.[56] And in the corporate sector, practitioners in the wellness movement have been concerned about the dearth of high quality, current information about their field.[57] More formal program evaluations would provide the needed cost-benefit analyses.

In spite of all that has been written about fitness in the last decade, there is still "widespread confusion" regarding its risks and benefits.[58] Among the most pervasive myths is one suggesting that in order to achieve the health benefits of exercise an individual must spend many hours exercising every week. The reality is that regular exercise does not have to take more than twenty to thirty minutes three days a week.[59] Even the medical profession has been chastized for not passing along to patients the good news about exercise. A doctor at Massachusetts General Hospital says that "exercise is one of the best kept secrets in preventive medicine" and that education about exercise is "insignificant" at most medical schools.[60] Evidently, there is a lack of communication within the medical community as well.

With the increase in knowledge related to fitness, the best information resource may not yet be in print. One example is a group of executives from fourteen San Francisco companies with wellness programs that gets together on a regular basis to trade information, to select and try experiments whose results are reported back to the group, and to swap information on vendors. This network efficiently generates and disseminates highly relevant information that might not be available any other way.[61] Although a general body of knowledge is available on fitness, the need has been documented for the more specific information required for tailoring fitness programs for individual applications.[62]

Market research in the fitness industry relies on national trend data combined with local data giving the specifics of the community — population, composition, resources, and other special characteristics. Unfortunately, reliable trend data are not readily available.[63] Even if the information has been compiled, it may not be available. Market studies, for instance, are often proprietary. Even if they are not, they can be too expensive for most users, especially libraries and schools.

Libraries are often maintained by associations and corporations to provide fitness/wellness information to their constituents. But a life insurance company in New England found that 60 percent of its employees were not readers and were not used to reading as a way of getting information.[64] In this case, collections of special interest magazines, audio and video tapes might be an effective alternative.

If the "fit body-cum-self" is perceived as an information-processing machine, "a machine which can correct and guide itself by means of an internal expert system,"[65] we must take care to avoid indigestion from obsolete, incomplete, or incomprehensible data.

ROLE OF ASSOCIATIONS

Professional associations serving the fitness industry and related areas often encourage and promote research activities in their fields. Data are then made available through their publications. Major associations generally produce one or more of the following: journals, magazines, newsletters, directories, handbooks, manuals, professional development books or videos, conference proceedings, and various special reports. Most associations support their profession by: providing leadership, conducting program evaluations, serving as an information clearinghouse, offering training and certification, and hosting annual conferences to report on industry developments.

Communities often use major health associations to assist in their health promotion activities. Local chapters of the American Lung Association, the American Heart Association, the American Cancer Society, and other national health-related groups frequently provide health promotion intervention at many sites. The YMCAs and YWCAs provide fitness programming and health promotion activities for all ages that are well-supervised and reasonably priced.

PROFESSIONAL PREPARATION

Fitness experts come with varied professional backgrounds and educational specializations. Students in undergraduate and graduate programs can specialize in such fields as exercise test technology, exercise physiology, and worksite health promotion.[66] And an increasing number of schools are offering courses and programs in adapted physical activity at both the undergraduate and graduate levels.

Departments offering fitness-related courses vary widely, from the traditional departments of physical education, health, physical education and recreation, or health education to others less familiar, such as the Department of Kinesiology at the University of Colorado, the Department of Human Kinetics and Leisure Studies at George Washington University, the Department of Fitness and Lifetime Sports at Pennsylvania College of Technology, the Department of Sport Fitness and Leisure Studies at Dean Junior College, and the Movement Science Department at Springfield College. These examples are taken from the *Physical Education Gold Book*,[67] which offers detailed information about physical education departments in American colleges and universities. Guides published by associations, organizations, and commercial publishers are the most direct source of information on schools offering professional preparation for fitness/wellness careers.[68] A review of the affiliations of contributing authors to books, journals, and proceedings will indicate leading institutions in these areas as will a review of schools mentioned consistently in the literature.

There is a growing demand for graduate degree programs in health, physical education, and recreation as a result of two trends: (1) an awareness of the influence of lifestyle factors on quality of life and (2) the growing cost of medical care. An overview of five well-known graduate programs indicates the varying degrees and specializations that are possible.[69]

Responding to the need for professional health/fitness managers for businesses, industries, and all levels of government, the American University instituted a Master of Science degree program in health/fitness management in 1980. The program design incorporates basic knowledge of business and managerial skills with scientific and clinical knowledge of exercise physiology, human biochemistry, psychology, and nutrition. Students in this program gain research and practical experience in the University's National Center for Health/Fitness.

The Department of Exercise Physiology at Illinois Benedictine College offers two degree programs leading to the Master of Science. The first is a program in exercise physiology with a specialization in preventive and rehabilitative cardiovascular health (PARCH). The second degree is in fitness management with an emphasis on the prevention of cardiovascular disease. Both programs are designed to conform with the established policies of the American College of Sports Medicine. Graduates are employed in the fields of cardiac rehabilitation and preventive medicine (mainly in a corporate fitness environment). The number of positions in corporate fitness are increasing rapidly so that the job market, especially in exercise physiology, is healthy.

Graduates of Northeastern University's Boston-Bouve College of Human Development Professions' health, sport, and leisure programs have diverse career options. Typical work settings include professional sports teams, corporate fitness programs, health clubs, hospital clinics, research laboratories, and recreational facilities. Classroom work in cardiovascular health and exercise may be combined with practical experience and sophisticated medical testing monitoring equipment in the university's Cardiovascular Health and Exercise Center.

Ohio State University offers individualized and specialized graduate programs taught by the graduate faculty of the School of Health, Physical Education, and Recreation. The five major sections of the school are Exercise Science and Special Populations, Health Education, Movement Arts and Outdoor Pursuits, Physical and Recreation Education, and Sport and Leisure Studies. Among its research facilities are a Teaching and Learning Laboratory and several exercise-science research laboratories.

The College of Health and Human Development at Pennsylvania State University focuses on the development of healthy individuals, prevention of illness, study of the processes leading to ill states and recovery after illness, and management of programs and service delivery systems. Seven programs offer graduate degrees through the college: Communication Disorders, Exercise and Sport Science, Health Education, Health Policy and Administration, Human Development and Family Studies, Nursing, and Recreation and Parks. In addition, the college houses three intercollege graduate programs: Genetics, Nutrition, and Physiology. Several research facilities, clinics, institutes, and laboratories are part of the college. Faculty research interests include heart disease, vitamin metabolism, aging, health care cost containment, and sports equipment design.

A notable training program for those considering careers in health promotion is the La Crosse Exercise and Health Program. Participants receive continuing education units (CEUs) from the University of Wisconsin, La Crosse, while continuing medical education units (CMUs) are provided through the Gunderson Medical Foundation.

Certification programs are both an alternative and a supplement to formal degrees in fitness and provide the basis for monitoring much of the professional preparation of fitness personnel. Several associations have established competency-based certification criteria for health and fitness professionals. The American College of Sports Medicine (ACSM) has prestigious programs for both rehabilitative and preventive track certifications. The ACSM preventive option was expanded in 1987 to include the following positions: (1) health fitness director, which requires a postgraduate degree in an allied health field or equivalent; (2) health fitness instructor; and (3) exercise leader/dance and exercise leader/fitness. Universities offering certification programs include: the University of Connecticut at Storrs, Adelphi University, Wake Forest University, the University of North Carolina at Charlottesville, and Pepperdine University.[70]

Mentioned frequently in discussions of fitness instructor certification is the Institute for Aerobics Research, founded by the renowned Dr. Kenneth Cooper, which provides certification workshops for fitness professionals in its Aerobic Center. These other associations are also setting new standards and certifying instructors: The International Dance Exercise Association (IDEA), the National Employee Services and Recreation Association (NESRA), the Universal Fitness Institute, and Jazzercise.

Such certifications appear among the credentials of fitness experts with traditional college degrees in health education, medicine, biology, leisure studies, and recreation. An example is fitness author Robert K. Cooper, whose educational preparation includes two doctorates — one in health education and one in health education and psychology — and certifications as a Health and Fitness Instructor from ACSM and as a Fitness Specialist from the Institute for Aerobics Research.

The increasing number of educational institutions and professional associations offering professional preparation for fitness personnel reflects society's growing awareness that a healthy lifestyle includes habitual physical activity.[71]

FITNESS FORECAST

John Naisbitt, in *Megatrends 2000*, predicts that an expanding concept of what it means to be human will characterize the twenty-first century.[72] As viewed by sociologists, the fitness movement is part of a larger movement of the "me generation" toward self-fulfillment.[73] Because fitness activities are frequently performed in a group, the body becomes a "focus of interaction" and a key constituent of the "me" or the experience of self in relation to the community.[74] Taken to its logical limit, this version of selfhood virtually equates the self with fitness activities.[75] In this context, "athletes and winners are looked up to as the new role models for the fitness lifestyle."[76] The popularity of exercise books and videos by film and sports celebrities supports this view.

The first phase of our current preoccupation with a healty lifestyle came in the early 1980s when Americans began to take increased responsibility for their health and the preventive approach toward medicine gained popularity. By the mid-1980s, consumer purchases of health food, health club memberships, workout videos, and fitness wear indicated that new health habits and awareness had become incorporated into everyday life.[77] In our current cultural environment, health is being transformed from a status — something one has — to an accomplishment — something one does.[78]

In the mid-1980s some fitness activities appeared to peak. Although reliable trend data is not available on fitness programs, there are some indications that participation declined in fitness programs outside the home in favor of in-home, schedule-flexible activities. The issue for the future is whether fitness will continue to be given a high priority in time and resource allocation by a population with limited amounts of both.[79]

In order to attract participants, fitness programs will have to respond to the needs of an increasingly diversified population.[80] Individualized fitness programs are recommended, especially for youth, the aged, and the disabled. Thomas Rowland, a pediatric cardiologist and author, has stressed the need for physical activity in childhood to prevent diseases later in life. During the 1980s, youth fitness benefited from major media attention to the link between physical activity, physical fitness, and positive health outcomes.[81] At the other end of the age range, a Gallup survey conducted for *American Health* magazine identified those over fifty as the fastest growing segment of exercise enthusiasts.[82] According to this poll, the share of people aged fifty and over who exercised regularly increased 46 percent between 1984 and 1986. Because the population will continue to age, more programs designed with decreased demands for physical competence are needed. Individualized exercise programs and workouts are also needed for those with some type of physical limitation. Adapted physical activities have proven social and economic benefits for the physically disabled.[83] The choice of a fitness program by the disabled is based on considerations shared by the able-bodied: effectiveness, cost, convenience, free time, attitudes, interests, and personality.[84]

Surveys have been conducted to determine which physical activities are the most popular. Participation in four activities—bicycling, camping, jogging, and tennis—have risen from limited popularity to the status of major pursuits over the past two decades, according to the 1982-83 *Nationwide Recreation Survey*.[85] Later surveys of 15,000 households by the Sporting Goods Manufacturers Association found that the fastest growing fitness activities were exercising with stair-climbing machines and treadmills.[86] And walking is now America's number one participation "sport" according to *Women's Sports and Fitness* magazine.[87]

Among all types of fitness participants, the 1980s' emphasis on "no pain, no gain" is being replaced by the relaxing workout. "The new exercise philosophy is to strive for total mind and body health." Fitness instructors and health clubs are combining ancient disciplines from the East, particularly yoga and t'ai chi, with Western exercises for "tough but mind-calming" routines.[88]

The fitness boom of the 1970s and early 1980s has been followed by a concurrent growth of interest in wellness. "A total wellness program is a marriage of fitness and good health practices."[89] As corporations continue to see the benefits in reduced health care costs, and increased employee productivity, employers are offering more and more programs to improve the physical condition of their employees. Estimates indicate that over half of all large American companies will provide wellness programs by 1995.[90]

Among the newest programming emphases in corporate wellness programs are prenatal education programs[91] and mental health programs, which bring the wisdom of psychology into the workplace.[92] Such programs reflect the broader definition of fitness that has evolved in the employee health movement.[93]

According to fitness industry experts, balance and moderation will be two key elements of fitness in the 1990s. Evidence from celebrity interviews and national surveys suggests that fitness will be increasingly integrated into everyday life and will be part of a person's family, relationships, and work.[94]

RATIONALE FOR
RESOURCE SELECTION

The intent of this chapter is to present a core collection of resources useful to initial research efforts, either cursory or in-depth. Because fitness is still evolving as a unique subject area, resources cited are multidisciplinary and have been taken from such related fields as sport, sports medicine, recreation, physical education, health, wellness, preventive medicine, psychology, and sociology. Sources included are appropriate for a variety of audience levels from scholarly to general interest. The current body of literature is not extensive compared to that of other more established leisure studies such as recreation, travel, and sport, so the intent has been to reflect the breath versus the depth of resources available. American sources are emphasized because Americans have been responsible for the fitness resurgence of the last two decades. Canadian contributions have been significant and have been included on a limited basis.

The annotated sources have been selected because they are generally available, current, comprehensive, critically acclaimed as significant to the subject, and/or offer unique information. A review of possible resources for this field suggests a need for additional works to support research, particularly bibliographies, conference proceedings, and statistical sources.

SOURCES

Guides and Handbooks

B-1. Chenoweth, David H. **Planning Health Promotion at the Worksite**. Indianapolis, IN: Benchmark. 1987.

Because Americans spend one-third of their lives at work, worksite health programs are a convenient way to promote an improved quality of life for all employees. Chenoweth has written a practical introduction to the basic concepts and activities employed by some of America's most successful worksite health promotion leaders. The intended audience is students and practicing professionals, but the book is also appropriate for the layperson needing background and resources on this topic. The book has three sections: planning health promotion, professionally preparing for corporate wellness programs, and appendices of cost-containment resources. The appendices are particularly valuable to those requiring additional information. A distinguishing feature is the number of tables, figures, models, resource lists, references, and other detailed information.

B-2. Dietrich, John, and Susan Waggoner. **Complete Health Club Handbook**. New York: Simon and Schuster, 1983.

For Americans considering beginning or renewing a health club membership, this guide assembles the information needed to select the most appropriate facility. In this essentially unregulated industry, consumers need objective information on what types of facilities are available, what types of social and recreational activities they offer, and how to evaluate the equipment and services being offered. Reviews are provided of more than 150 health clubs in ten major American cities. Appendices allow readers to locate major fitness centers in their state as well as various equipment manufacturers. A detailed index is included. This is a useful resource for both public and academic libraries.

B-3.   Glover, Bob, and Jack Shepherd. **The Family Fitness Handbook**. New York: Penguin, 1989.

A well-known fitness expert describes his physical fitness program for children. Parents and teachers are given a guide for improving the fitness level of children using a variety of practical and enjoyable activities. Most of the research and concepts for the book were a result of Glover's work with his son and his son's school physical education program. The book is designed primarily for children between the ages of five and twelve. Guidelines for preschoolers and teenagers are also discussed. Current, practical information is given on a wide range of fitness topics including family fitness evaluation tests, imaginative fitness games, special guidelines for girls and women, nutrition, and incorporating sports in a fitness program. The appendix section provides concise yet comprehensive listings of leading fitness organizations, programs, publishers, magazines, and newsletters. A detailed index allows the reader quick access to topics of interest.

B-4.   Paciorek, Michael J., and Jeffery A. Jones. **Sport and Recreation for the Disabled: A Resource Handbook**. Indianapolis, IN: Benchmark, 1989.

The growing interest in sports and recreation for those with disabilities has created a need for information on ways that people with disabilities can access sport and recreational opportunities. Hundreds of sources and individuals were consulted in the preparation of this text. Fifty-three sport and recreational activities are discussed for eight major disability groups. There is also a chapter on fitness programs. All chapters include: an activity overview, adapted equipment, equipment suppliers and manufacturers, additional resources, references, and suggested readings for those involved in research. Other features to recommend this text are numerous illustrations and photographs as well as the useful appendices. This resource is appropriate for anyone serving or providing information to the disabled.

B-5.   **Planning Facilities for Athletics, Physical Education and Recreation**. North Palm Beach, FL: Athletic Institute, and Reston, VA: American Alliance for Health, Physical Education, Recreation, and Dance, 1985.

There have been fourteen printings of this guide since its first publication in 1946. Interest in facility planning and construction is due to the increased leisure time in our society and a growing realization that physical activity is essential to the well-being of youth and adults. Architects and leading authorities in planning facilities for schools, colleges, municipalities, industry, military, and private clubs have contributed to this edition. Updated facility planning and construction has been included as well as expanded sections for certain program areas such as planning for the handicapped. References and illustrations abound and support the comprehensive text coverage of indoor, outdoor, swimming pool, stadium, and service area design.

B-6.   **Stanford Health and Exercise Handbook**. Champaign, IL: Leisure Press, 1989.

Readers are encouraged to celebrate the human body as the greatest high-tech invention of all time and to protect it from poor lifestyle habits. Exercise is presented as the key to achieving and maintaining optimum health for as long as possible. Successful strategies for health promotion and disease prevention used at the Stanford Center for Research in Disease Prevention are explained. The eight benefits to health that exercise provides are stressed: improved cardiovascular health, weight control, reduced serum cholesterol, lowered blood sugar, lowered blood pressure, increased bone density, psychological enhancement, and compressed morbidity. Contributing authors include specialists in cardiology, orthopedics, epidemiology, lipid biochemistry, nutrition, psychiatry, psychology, internal medicine, exercise physiology, and sports medicine. This is a good introduction to major fitness concepts presented in an extremely palatable style—complete with cartoons.

B-7. **The Stanford Health and Exercise Program**. Champaign, IL: Leisure Press, 1989.

This videotape, produced to be used alone or as a companion to the *Stanford Health and Exercise Handbook*, summarizes the benefits of exercise and presents four fitness self-assessment tests and the Stanford Workout. During the workout segment, three low-impact aerobic workouts—for beginning, intermediate, and advanced levels—are demonstrated simultaneously. This is intriguing, but it takes some practice to follow the workout level of your choice. At the end of the video, five world-class athletes and former Olympians show how to prepare for participation in their sports.

Noteworthy Books

B-8. Cooper, Kenneth H. **Aerobics**. New York: Bantam, 1969.

Touted on the cover as the "world's most popular physical fitness program," this is a seminal work in the field. Dr. Cooper's physical fitness plan was the first to scientifically measure how much exercise was enough to maintain a healthy body. His approach was to take the popular forms of activity and measure the amounts of energy expended so that anyone could select one and know how much exercise would be necessary for a beneficial effect. Dr. Cooper popularized the concept of "aerobic" exercises (literally, those "with oxygen"), which demand considerable oxygen, supplied from the heart and lungs, and which can be continued for long periods of time.

The book was based on four years' study of thousands of men to determine the relationship of physical fitness to health. Even in the 1960s it was called "a major contribution to a healthier America" (preface). The original work caused a revolution in physical fitness training and practice. Subsequently, millions of copies have been sold in various printings.

B-9. Cooper, Robert K. **Health and Fitness Excellence**. Boston: Houghton Mifflin, 1989.

Described as a "scientific action plan," this book is based on the latest discoveries about fitness, diet, stress, and other self-care priorities. The author is a health professional, teacher, researcher, and athlete who has gathered the self-care ideas of hundreds of scientists, physicians, psychologists, educators, and other experts worldwide and grouped them in seven key areas: stress strategies, exercise options, nutritional wellness, body fat control, postural vitality, rejuvenation, and mind and life unity. This program is based on the "positive wellness" concept of health, the idea that the major determinants of health, fitness, and longevity are the personal choices made by each individual. Because the large amount of information is organized into short chapters where key concepts are highlighted, the reader is not overwhelmed. Further assistance to the reader is provided by an extensive index, chapter notes, and a resources list of relevant periodicals. This is an excellent synthesis of current health and fitness literature for health-conscious individuals, educators, executives, and parents.

B-10. Garrick, James G., and Peter Radetsky. **Be Your Own Personal Trainer**. New York: Crown, 1989.

As the title implies, this is an example of an individualized personal fitness guide. The author has twenty-five years' experience as a sports medicine physician. The chapters are intended to be read and followed in sequence. They cover practical approaches to fitness assessment; goal-setting; training for sports activities; and working out for strength, endurance, and flexibility. The index is in-depth for the scope of the book, but there are no references. This is a good initial resource for the layperson interested in starting a fitness routine.

B-11. Getchell, Bud. **The Fitness Book**. Indianapolis, IN: Benchmark, 1987.

Getchell presents the National Institute for Fitness and Sport's position on the importance of exercise in everyday life. The basic steps for developing an overall fitness program are outlined in an easy-to-follow format. Chapters are concise and include a summary section, which reinforces concepts presented. Numerous figures and tables supplement the text throughout. Outstanding features include a detailed table of contents and an index.

B-12. Green, Harvey. **Fit for America: Health, Fitness, Sport and American Society**. Baltimore, MD: Johns Hopkins University Press, 1988.

This work discusses and documents both the continuity and change in the ways Americans have thought about good health throughout modern history. The focus is on the perceptions and actions of Americans from the 1830s to the 1980s. Many surprising facts emerge, including the insight that "we of the last quarter of the twentieth century did not invent aerobics, weight-lifting, exercise machines, 'health' foods, or the variety of other ways we employ [today] to attain the bodily state we desire" (preface).

This study explores the "ideas, realities, and the solutions" middle class Americans have had to the problems of health and fitness for over a century. The sources investigated included catalogs, advertisements, diaries, letters, journals, artifacts, professional texts, athletic instructional manuals, advice books, and household guides. The book is both scholarly in presentation and entertaining in delivery. Numerous photographs of the varied source materials enrich the text. There are extensive reference notes on each chapter for the interested researcher, but chapters remain highly readible for the layperson. An index aids access to specific areas of interest. This study was supported both by the Strong Museum and the National Endowment for the Humanities.

B-13. Grover, Kathryn. **Fitness in American Culture: Images of Health, Sport, and the Body, 1830-1940**. Baltimore, MD: Margaret Woodbury Strong Museum, 1990.

This book is a good companion volume to Green's *Fit for America* (entry B-12) and presents six essays on popular views of health and fitness from the time period covered. Both books are appropriate for college libraries.

B-14. Rippe, James M. **Dr. James M. Rippe's Fit for Success: Proven Strategies for Executive Health**. New York: Prentice-Hall, 1989.

This is the first major summary of health and fitness attitudes and practices among top executives. Over 1,000 executives were surveyed. As a group, they were found to take regular exercise seriously and to be concerned about their health. In addition to the study results, source materials for the book included current medical and scientific literature and the clinical experiences of Rippe and his colleagues. Among the chapter topics are: exercise and cardiovascular health, setting up an individual exercise program, nutrition and weight control, stress management, daily lifestyle impact on health, establishing corporate fitness programs, and executive visions and philosophies related to health and fitness. Two appendices are included: one is the survey questionnaire and a brief description of the methodology; the other is the identity of the forty CEOs interviewed for the study. Chapter references and an index are included.

B-15. Rowland, Thomas W. **Exercise and Children's Health**. Champaign, IL: Human Kinetics, 1990.

Written by a pediatric cardiologist with an extensive research background, this book "endeavors to paint a broad picture of the role of exercise in children's health" (preface). It can aid parents, physicians, clinicians, researchers, teachers, and students in helping youngsters grow into healthy adults. Three major content areas are defined: developmental exercise physiology, the influence of exercise on health, and strategies for improving the exercise habits of children. The book's hands-on guidelines are for healthy children and for those with special health problems like obesity, heart disease, asthma, diabetes, and seizure disorders. Other features of the book include an appendix of patient guidelines for specific activities, a reference section for readers needing more comprehensive information, and ample photographs, figures, and tables to enhance the text. Overall, the real value of the books may be its "persuasive evidence that the promotion of physical activity in young individuals is a valuable effort that can pay significant long-term health dividends" (preface).

B-16. Sharkey, Brian J. **Physiology of Fitness**. 3d ed. Champaign, IL: Human Kinetics, 1990.

This "thinking person's fitness book" is intended for interested laypersons and enthusiastic professionals who need the latest findings about the relationship between exercise and cardiovascular health, dieting and the "yo-yo" effect, strength training, aerobic tests, low back fitness, eating disorders, and fat intake. The book is divided into five parts that correspond to major dimensions of fitness: aerobic, muscular, weight control, health, and lifestyle. Chapters under each division facilitate learning by beginning with a list of objectives, highlighting key information, and illustrating key concepts with numerous tables and figures. A useful feature is 100 pages of appendices with practical approaches to topics including fitness testing, health risk analysis, principles of training, and weight control. This fitness guide has been refined over three editions to reflect ongoing research on all dimensions of fitness: the physiological, the psychological, and the mystical.

B-17. Shephard, Roy J. **Fitness in Special Populations**. Champaign, IL: Human Kinetics, 1990.

Designed to address the need for "a clear, synthetic account of the current fitness status of the disabled and their responses to vigorous, competitive physical activity" (p. viii), this book is a compilation of research on fitness assessment, programming, and performance for people with various forms of physical disabilities, including mental retardation. Ten chapters cover critical issues such as disability classification, methods of quantitative assessment, response to training programs, social difficulties faced by the handicapped, and the concerns of key international organizations. Appendices feature other texts in adapted physical education, norms for fitness tests, integration guidelines, and a glossary of simplified medical terms. A comprehensive, sixty-two page bibliography of current research is an important feature. The suggested audience is senior undergraduate and graduate students in physical education and physiotherapy and other health professionals involved in exercise and training programs for disabled persons.

Dissertations

B-18.   Chamberland, Craig, and Robert J. Moffatt, eds. **Completed Research in Health, Physical Education, Recreation and Dance**. vol. 31. Reston, VA: American Alliance for Health, Physical Education, Recreation and Dance, 1989.

This compilation covers master's and doctoral theses completed in 1988 in the subjects of health, physical education, recreation, dance, and allied areas. It is arranged in three parts. The first section is a subject index in alphabetical order. In the second section, theses abstracts are numbered in alphabetical order according to institution. Finally, a bibliography lists published research in relevant periodicals. Any university or college is invited to submit abstracts of theses for review and possible inclusion. This is a good starting point to locate fitness or employee fitness theses, especially those on the master's level.

B-19.   **Dissertation Abstracts International**. Ann Arbor, MI: University Microfilms, 1938- . Online and CD-ROM formats available.

This source is invaluable in tracking down dissertations published on the topics of fitness and health. Thirty-five thousand citations from more than 500 institutions are indexed here annually. Author and keyword indexes are provided. (See entries A-37, C-18, and D-13.)

B-20.   **Health, Physical Education and Recreation Microform Publications Bulletin**. Eugene, OR: University of Oregon, 1949- . 5 issues/yr.

Bibliographic data and abstracts of master's and doctoral theses from U.S. universities are recorded on microfilm. Among the topics available are physical fitness, employee health programs, and physical education and training. (See entry C-19.)

Bibliographies

B-21.   **Physical Fitness/Sports Medicine**. Washington, DC: President's Council on Physical Fitness and Sports. 1978- . Quarterly.

A bibliography of citations from over 3,000 selected periodicals retrieved by computer from the MEDLARS database of the National Library of Medicine. Included are foreign-language periodicals with English abstracts. Selected papers from conference proceedings are also included. Access is provided via subject and author indexes. A listing of serials indexed is provided at the end. This bibliography is inexpensive and comprehensive for intermediate and advanced levels of research reports. A "best buy" for interested individuals or institutions.

B-22.   **Sport Bibliography**. Champaign, IL: Human Kinetics, 1986- . Annual.

The Sport Information Resource Centre (SIRC) describes itself as "the largest resource centre in the world collecting and disseminating information in the area of sport, physical education, physical fitness and sports medicine" (preface). This series of bibliographies is produced from data in their SPORT online database (entry B-43). Each focuses on a specific topic and contains approximately 200 bibliographic references. Bibliographies are bilingual, English and French only. Titles are updated and added as required. Those related to health and fitness are: *Physical Fitness in the Third Age*, *Physical Activity and Mental Health*, *Employee Fitness*, *Nutrition and Physical Activity*, and *Sport and Recreation for the Disabled: A Bibliography 1984-1990* (see entry C-25). In addition to bibliographic data, citations contain a research level rating: basic, intermediate, or advanced. Abstracts are generally provided for research reports and for intermediate or technical material. The bibliographies are informative, inexpensive, and produced by a respected information source. (See entry C-24.)

Dictionaries and Encyclopedias

B-23. Cureton, Thomas K., ed. **Human Performance: Efficiency and Improvements in Sports, Exercise and Fitness**, vol. 4 of *Encyclopedia of Physical Education, Fitness, and Sports*. Reston, VA: American Alliance for Health, Physical Education, Recreation and Dance, 1985.

This volume of the *Encyclopedia of Physical Education, Fitness, and Sports* (see entry C-31) emphasizes the benefits obtained by the consistent participation in the sports and exercise activities described in the previous three volumes. Volume 4 takes widely scattered research and restates it in simplified terms so that research results are more comprehensible to the general reader. Rather than merely describing the sports and exercises, the evidence summarized focuses on their "anatomical, physiological, and psychological effects on adults" (preface). Results are organized into nine sections with varying numbers of essays by leaders in the field. Brief biographies of these section contributors are found in a biographical appendix included with this volume. Researchers will be pleased with the comprehensive references that accompany each essay.

B-24. **Encyclopedia of Business Information Sources**. with **Supplement**. Edited by James Woy. 7th ed. Detroit: Gale Research, 1989.

B-25. **Encyclopedia of Health Information Sources**. Detroit: Gale Research, 1989.

These two Gale Research encyclopedias effectively meet the information needs of executives and managers searching for background information on a wide variety of health-related topics as well as specific information on a particular subject. Although the primary audience is business administrators, others who might benefit from these two resources are librarians, researchers, analysts, planners, and others needing information on business-related subjects. A *Supplement* accompanies the first title and includes fifty new topics and revised coverage of twenty seventh-edition topics. Among the new topics is employee wellness. A related entry is the health care industry. Among the sources of information covered for these topics are: directories, periodicals and newsletters, research centers and institutes, trade associations, and professional societies.

B-26. Friedberg, Ardy. **The Facts on File Dictionary of Fitness**. New York: Facts on File, 1984.

The "new world of fitness" jargon and popular phrases borrowed from the world of athletes, coaches, doctors, and nutritionists are the province of this reference book. Words selected for inclusion represent "the essential elements of an adequate fitness vocabulary." Word arrangement is alphabetical with cross-references provided for convenience. An advantage is longer definitions of fitness-related terms than are found in less specialized dictionaries.

Directories

B-27. Association for Fitness in Business. **Annual Information Directory and Resource Guide**. Stamford, CT: Association for Fitness in Business. Annual.

The Association for Fitness in Business (AFB) membership includes professionals from many disciplines — business, education, medicine, psychology — working together to encourage lifestyle strategies that lead to improved health and well-being. They also share the conviction that worksite fitness programs result in reduced health care costs. The *Directory* is designed to serve as an educational and networking resource for AFB members and other fitness professionals. It is also a convenient reference for the identification and selection of fitness-related products and services such as consultants, associations, schools, and internships. This is an expensive, specialized resource most feasible for large academic or special libraries serving this population.

B-28. **The ... Directory: Exercise and Physical Fitness Programs**. Omaha, NE: American Business Directories. Annual.

Compiled from *The Yellow Pages*, this directory features over 7,000 listings complete with name, address, phone number, franchise/speciality information, and Yellow Page advertisement specifics organized alphabetically by state. Completely updated each year, the directory information is taken from more than 4,800 Yellow Page telephone directories throughout the United States. It is a specialized reference tool useful for marketing research information.

B-29. **Health Information Resources in the Federal Government**. 4th ed. Washington, DC: Office of Disease Prevention and Health Promotion, National Health Information Center, 1987.

This very inexpensive directory identifies federal and federally sponsored health information resources. The user is directed to a central information source for each agency or department cited, and complete purchase information is included. Among the categories of resources covered are: federal programs and policies, Office of Disease Prevention and Health Promotion (ODPHP) monographs, community, worksite and school health promotion programs, nutrition, professional education, educational materials, and other sources. This is a handy resource for anyone handling inquiries concerning health matters.

B-30. **Physical Education Gold Book 1987-89**. Champaign, IL: Human Kinetics, 1987.

This is the only directory of physical education professionals in higher education. It is intended as an "everyday handbook" for information on physical education departments and individuals. Over 6,000 individuals at 590 two-year and four-year institutions are listed. Part 1 includes information on prominent physical education programs. Part 2, the bulk of the publication, provides individual faculty listings. In this section, faculty may indicate their three major areas of interest from among over eighty possible aspects of physical education. A weakness of the publication is the lack of information provided by some respondents. This is a needed resource at a very reasonable price and should be of value to practitioners, educators, administrators, vendors, and researchers.

Indexes, Abstracts, and Databases

B-31.   **ABI/Inform**. Louisville, KY: UMI Data Courier, 1971- . Weekly updates. Online and CD-ROM formats available.

A primary database to identify articles on corporate wellness programs and exercise/physical fitness activities in the corporate sector. The database indexes and abstracts articles from nearly 800 business and management periodicals. It provides online coverage similar to the print coverage offered by the *Business Periodicals Index* (entries B-34 and D-22). (See entry D-19.)

B-32.   **Ageline**. Washington, DC: American Association of Retired Persons, 1978- . Bimonthly updates. Available online.

This bibliographic database identifies journal, book, book chapter, and report information on social gerontology. The database is built primarily on the library collection of the AARP's National Gerontology Resource Center, which collects aging-related publications from trade publishers and organizational sources. Those interested in elder fitness will benefit from its coverage of health-related concerns including health care services and costs, mental and physical health assessment, nutrition and exercise, theories of aging, and services for older adults. There is no equivalent print index for this database.

B-33.   **A-V Online**. Albuquerque, NM: 1964- . Quarterly updates. Available online.

This is the online version of the National Information Center for Educational Media (NICEM) print indexes. The database identifies nonprint educational media for all levels of education from preschool to postgraduate in all academic areas. Professional development and teacher training resources are included. The following media are included: 16mm films, filmstrips, overhead transparencies, videotapes, audiotapes, motion cartridges, slides, and slide sets. Health education and physical education are heavily covered subject areas.

B-34.   **Business Periodicals Index**. New York: H. W. Wilson, 1958- . Monthly, except August, with bimonthly, semiannual, and annual cumulations. Online and CD-ROM formats available.

This is a first-choice resource for aspects of fitness and wellness in the industrial or corporate sector. Over 300 major English language business magazines are indexed. Another advantage of this index is its widespread availability in libraries. (See entry D-22.)

B-35.   **Consumer Health and Nutrition Index**. Phoenix, AZ: Oryx, 1985- . Quarterly.

The purpose of this index is to give the layperson access to significant articles in popular health and general magazines and newsletters. Consumers, practitioners, and libraries have a single source for accessing scattered sources of information on subjects such as nutrition, particular diseases, alternative medicine, drugs, exercise, the disabled, women's health, child care, and natural health products. The focus in on practical health concerns, and articles are taken from over ninety periodicals and nine newsletters. Subject headings have subdivisions for "Personal Accounts," "Statistics," "Law and Legislation," and "Book Reviews." Citations include special notes to alert the user if an article is an editorial, letter to the editor, abstract, review, or very short piece. The number of references is also noted. An impressive reference tool that lives up to its goal of being "one-stop access" to popular health literature at an affordable price.

B-36.   **Consumer Reports**. Mount Vernon, NY: Consumers Union, 1982- . Monthly updates. Available online.

This full-text database contains articles and product recalls from the eleven regular monthly issues of *Consumer Reports* magazine and the twelve monthly issues of two newsletters, *Consumer Reports Travel Letter* and *Consumer Reports Health Letter*. In addition to product testing results in the health area, *Consumer Reports* also provides articles on health, medical matters, and nutrition. The *Consumer Reports Health Letter* is intended to give objective and reliable guidance on health care management from experts in health and medicine. Information is provided to assist readers in making decisions about health care services and products. Full-text reports cover topics such as diet, exercise, fitness, nutrition, and important medical developments.

B-37.   **Current Index to Journals in Education (CIJE)**. Phoenix, AZ: Oryx, 1969- . Monthly, with cumulative annual index. Online and CD-ROM formats available.

For articles on fitness, health education, and physical education, this index—also referred to as the *CIJE*—is an essential reference. A typical issue indexes approximately 1,500 articles from nearly 800 journals. Alternate formats include microfiche to depository libraries and online and CD-ROM as the ERIC database. Most libraries supporting education or teacher-training programs will provide access to some format of this index. (See entry A-52.)

B-38.   **Education Index**. New York: H. W. Wilson, 1929- . Monthly (except July and August), with quarterly and annual cumulations. Online and CD-ROM formats available.

This index is recommended as a companion to the *CIJE* for coverage of all levels of education. There is enough difference in coverage to recommend consulting both indexes for a comprehensive research effort. *Education Index* is also available online as WILSONLINE and on CD-ROM as WILSONDISC. This index is commonly found in moderate to large public and academic libraries. (See entry A-53.)

B-39.   **Educational Film and Video Locator**. 4th ed. New York: R. R. Bowker, 1990.

This index brings together 51,900 entries for educational films and videos. The titles listed have been compiled from the forty-six media collections belonging to members of the Consortium of College and University Media Centers. Users may access information by subject, title, and series. Over 600 subjects are listed. Physical fitness is among the current topical issues added to this updated fourth edition. To identify rental sources, holdings identifiers are included in each entry.

B-40. **Educational Resources Information Center (ERIC)**. Washington, DC: Affiliated with the U.S. Office of Education, Office of Educational Research and Improvement, 1966- . Monthly updates. Online and CD-ROM formats available.

With over 700,000 citations, ERIC is the largest education database in the world. Sponsored by the U.S. Department of Education, Office of Educational Research and Improvement (OERI), its citations cover research documents, journal articles, technical reports, program descriptions and evaluations, and curricular materials in the field of education. The database is a comprehensive source for physical and health education information. Students, teachers, librarians, researchers, parents, administrators, and the general public would be appropriate users. Its print counterparts are *Resources in Education* (RIE) (entry A-58) and *Current Index to Journals in Education* (entry A-52). (See entry A-54.)

B-41. National Information Center for Educational Media (NICEM). **Film and Video Finder**. 2d ed. Medford, NJ: Plexus, 1989.

NICEM indexes have provided librarians, media specialists, and teachers with bibliographic guides to educational media since 1964. This latest film and video index has 110,000 entries. Entry content and arrangement is similar to Bowker's *Locator*. NICEM also has indexes to filmstrips, audiocassettes, transparencies, slide sets, and other nonprint materials. Separate, more subject-specific, indexes available from NICEM include: *Coaches Guide to Sports Audiovisuals* and *Wellness Media*.

B-42. **Physical Education Index**. Cape Girardeau, MO: Ben Oak, 1978- . Quarterly, with the fourth issue a bound hardcover cumulation.

This subject index provides comprehensive coverage of domestic and foreign periodicals published in English. Preference is given to articles on dance, health, physical education, physical therapy, recreation, sports, and sports medicine. Also covered are more specific topics such as physical fitness, biomechanics-kinesiology, research, and training. Book reviews are a separate section in the back of each issue. (See entry C-48.)

B-43. **SPORT**. Gloucester, Canada: Sport Information Resource Centre, 1949- . Monthly updates. Available online.

This is an international bibliographic database covering all aspects of sport, fitness, and recreation. SPORT includes both practical and research information. Among the fitness-related subjects covered are: physical education, exercise physiology, motor learning, and physical fitness. Information sources include sport and medical journals, books, book chapters, conference proceedings, theses, reports, and other monographs. To assist users, each document is classified according to intended audience level, from basic to advanced. The print counterpart is *SportSearch* (entry C-53).

Core Journals

B-44. **Adapted Physical Activity Quarterly**. Champaign, IL: Human Kinetics, 1984- . Quarterly. Indexed in *Physical Education Index*, *PsycINFO*, and *SportSearch*.

A multidisciplinary approach is employed in the study of physical activities for special populations by this scholarly journal. Research from such disciplines as health care, occupational therapy, physical education, physical therapy, recreation, rehabilitation, and gerontology is highlighted. The latest theoretical and applied research related to adaptations of equipment, activity, facilities, methodology, and/or setting are discussed. Articles are selected for inclusion based on a panel's judgment of their scholarship and relevance. New book and media reviews are a regular feature. This journal is recommended for professional collections and libraries in institutions with physical education programs. (See entry C-50.)

B-45. **American Fitness**. Sherman Oaks, CA: Aerobics and Fitness Association of America, 1987- . 9 issues/yr. Indexed in *Physical Education Index*.

Fitness professionals and advocates will find this a highly readable magazine covering aerobic exercise, sports, fitness, and health topics. Feature articles are varied and of interest to a wide audience, including consumers, instructors, club owners, and others involved with the fitness industry. Regular columns cover nutrition, resorts, and travel news. Departments cover fitness news, trends, and research. The "Product Shopper" lists companies providing products and services to the fitness community and includes useful lists of books, media, and associations. A subject index to articles in previous issues is published periodically. This is a good, basic purchase for libraries and individuals needing to know more about aerobics and fitness than general popular-interest magazines can provide. (Formerly called *Aerobics and Fitness*.)

B-46. **American Health: Fitness of Body and Mind**. New York: American Health Partners, 1982- . Monthly (except February and August). Indexed in *Readers' Guide to Periodical Literature*, *Abridged Readers' Guide*, *Consumer Health Nutrition Index*, and *Readers' Guide Abstracts*.

More popular than scholarly in approach, this journal is a good starting point for background information and an overview of health-related topics. The audience would be someone wanting more than a general interest magazine and less than a professional journal. Feature articles cover nutrition, medicine, fitness and athletics, prevention, and psychology. The "News to Use" section has updates on fitness, nutrition, and medical happenings.

B-47. **American Journal of Health Promotion: AJHP**. Rochester Hills, MI: American Journal of Health Promotion, 1986- . Bimonthly. Indexed in *Hospital Literature Index* and *Human Resources Abstracts*.

This is the official journal for members of the Association for Fitness in Business. Articles are abstracted, illustrated with tables and figures, and referenced. They contain research evaluation methods and results with discussion by experts in the field. Scholarly, yet readable for the layperson, this journal usefully interprets research findings from journals aimed at the health professional such as the *American Journal of Preventive Medicine*, the *Journal of the American Medical Association*, and the *American Journal of Public Health*.

B-48. **American Journal of Public Health: APH**. Washington, DC: American Public Health Association, 1971- . Monthly. Widely indexed and abstracted, in such indexes as *Index Medicus*, *Social Science Index*, *Hospital Literature Index*, *Physical Education Index*, *Leisure, Recreation and Tourism Abstracts*, *CIJE*, and *SportSearch*.

This is a peer-reviewed journal that publishes original research and studies in forty-five public disciplines. Articles are scholarly in tone and format. The abstracts preceding each article are useful for the non-public health professional who wishes to keep current with developments in fitness research without doing in-depth reading. References follow each article for those who wish to consult additional sources. The "Book Corner" reviews recently published books and classifies them by subject matter. Selected titles are described in detailed annotations. Although fitness is only one of many topics covered by the journal, it is a source of research often cited elsewhere in the literature.

B-49. **Business and Health**. Oradell, NJ: Medical Economics, 1983- . Monthly (except combined January/Feburary and July/August). Indexed in *Hospital Literature Index*, *Current Literature on Aging*, and *Work Related Abstracts*.

This journal is designed for employers interested in corporate health care policy and cost management strategies. Written from the business perspective, the content is more informative than scholarly. Each issue contains special reports on critical health issues, in-depth feature articles by experts in the field, and regular columns providing updates on legislation, regulations, current developments, trends, innovations, and controversies. The most appreciative audiences would be those involved in corporate wellness, personnel, health care, and elder care.

B-50. **Corporate Fitness**. Santa Monica, CA: Brentwood, 1987- . Bimonthly (with an extra issue in February). Indexing information not available. Under the former title of *Corporate Fitness and Recreation*, it was indexed in *Physical Education Index*.

Subtitled "The Journal for Employee Health and Services Programs," this journal is directed to administrators of corporate health-promotion programs, corporate medical directors, and wellness programs. Readers do not require any particular subject area background. Subjects are topical and oriented toward the practitioner. Regular features include the "Industry Pulse"—news, trends, events, and product reports—and a "Spotlight" on equipment news. An annual buyers' guide lists equipment, products, and services offered by hundreds of companies for facility planning, fitness/strength/conditioning, health and wellness, and off-site fitness.

B-51. **Journal of Physical Education, Recreation and Dance**. Reston, VA: American Alliance for Health, Physical Education, Recreation and Dance, 1981- . Monthly, except July, with November/December and May/June issues combined. Indexed in *CIJE*, *Exceptional Child Education Resources*, *Media Review Digest*, *Physical Education Index*, *SportSearch*, and *Education Index*.

Professional educators at all levels rely on this journal for articles on current issues, new methods, trends, and materials in physical education and the related fields of recreation and dance. It reports on developments in Canada as well as the United States. Coverage is also given to physical education concerns of the disabled. Among the regular features are: letters, research reports, teaching tips, news, reviews, new books, and products. An essential subscription for any institution with teacher-preparation programs in physical education. (See entry C-51.)

B-52. **Journal of the International Council for Health, Physical Education, and Recreation**. Reston, VA: International Council for Health, Physical Education, and Recreation, 1988- . Quarterly. Indexed in *CIJE*, *Physical Education Index*, and *SportSearch*.

This is the official journal of the International Council for Health, Physical Education, and Recreation (ICHPER), specializing in topics of interest to an international audience of teachers and those who serve the teaching profession. It is a refereed journal and articles are scholarly in format. Preference is given to articles dealing with applications and implications for the practitioner in regular and special education. Research studies are selected for coverage that suggests ways to improve programs and activities. Information is also included on print and nonprint resources, conferences and congresses, and world happenings of the ICHPER.

B-53.   **Prevention**. Emmaus, PA: Rodale, 1950- . Monthly. Indexed in both popular and scholarly sources including *Readers' Guide to Periodical Literature*, *Abridged Readers' Guide*, *Magazine Index*, *Popular Magazine Review*, and *Chemical Abstracts*.

Billing itself as "America's leading health magazine," *Prevention* is among the major magazines advocating a preventive and participatory approach to health care. The magazine is for the lay reader and presents current developments in health in an easy-to-read and understand format. Articles by medical experts cover a wide range of topics, including women's health, dental health, nutritional medicine, weight loss programs, pet care, holistic medicine, and fitness/exercise benefits. The "Mailbag" department has both letters to the editor from readers offering testimonials to the value of advice garnered from the magazine and "home remedies" for all kinds of health conditions. The magazine's advertisements are a good source for information about health products and services. The "Healthfront" section offers medical news and "feel-better tips." This magazine should have wide appeal for homes, libraries, schools, doctors' offices, and corporations with wellness programs or aspirations.

B-54.   **Quest**. Champaign, IL: Human Kinetics, 1963- . 3 issues/yr. Indexed in *CIJE*, *Education Index*, and *Women Studies Abstracts*.

Sponsored by the National Association for Physical Education in Higher Education, this is a professional development journal concerned with critical issues for physical educators at this level. Although original research is not published by the journal, articles are solicited that are based on current research. Both theoretical and practical articles are printed. Journal readership includes academicians, teachers, and administrators.

B-55.   **Self**. New York: Conde Nast, 1979- . Monthly. Indexed in *Popular Magazine Review* and *Consumer Health and Nutrition Index*.

Designed for the contemporary woman interested in total mind-body awareness, this popular magazine offers guidance on sex, fashion, fitness, coping, nutrition, money management, and beauty. Behind its slick packaging, the magazine does contain worthwhile articles by contributors whose credentials are given, articles reprinted from reputable sources like *Science* magazine, and articles adapted from popular books. Lots of useful information based on research reports, surveys, government studies, and assorted sources can be found in the "News" sections. Readers will probably be women who might not get this information in a more academic magazine.

Conference Proceedings

B-56.   American Academy of Physical Education. **Physical Activity and Aging**, vol. 22 of The Academy Papers. Champaign, IL: Human Kinetics, 1989.

Conference proceedings of the academy are published annually and address a topic of current importance to the membership and others interested in physical education. Each publication in the series is notable for a scholarly approach featuring contributions from subject specialists in the field, extensive chapter references, research results supported by statistical data, and suggestions for further research. In this issue on aging, educators from fourteen universities are represented. The concern with maintaining fitness to age sixty-five and over comes from the knowledge that this is the fastest-growing age group in our society. This volume seeks to clarify the benefits, risks, and parameters of physical activity for our aging population. The newest title in this series, volume 23, is *The Evolving Undergraduate Major*.

B-57.   Bouchard, Claude, et al., eds. **Exercise, Fitness, and Health: A Consensus of Current Knowledge**. Champaign, IL: Human Kinetics, 1990.

An impressive amount of research is covered in this volume of sixty-two papers from eighty-seven internationally known exercise scientists. This is a "first-ever" consensus statement developed as a result of presentations at the 1988 International Conference on Exercise, Fitness, and Health held in Toronto, Canada. Papers presented are based on the assumption that "there are complex relationships between the levels of habitual physical activity, physical and physiological fitness, and health" (introduction). A highly recommended resource for academic libraries as well as for its intended audience of physical educators, exercise scientists, sports medicine specialists, and health care professionals.

B-58.   Gisolfi, Carl V., and David R. Lamb, eds. **Youth, Exercise, and Sport**, vol. 2 of Perspectives in Exercise Science and Sports Medicine. Indianapolis, IN: Benchmark, 1989.

This volume is part of a series of annual conference proceedings sponsored by the Quaker Oats Company, which donates all royalties from the series to the American College of Sports Medicine Foundation. International experts review the current research in their subjects and present the results in a detailed yet readable style. Each paper contributed is subjected to expert review and discussion by conference participants. This discussion is included in the chapter. Volume 2 targets important issues relating to the fitness of children but includes literature on youths up to the age of eighteen. Chapter outlines and summary sections highlight key points and are especially helpful for the interested layperson. Currently, there are three other volumes in this series dealing with prolonged exercise, fluid homeostasis during exercise, and ergogenics (performance enhancement).

Statistical Sources/Trend Data

B-59.   **American Demographics**. Ithaca, NY: American Demographics, 1979- . Monthly (except bimonthly July/August).

This magazine is as at home on the newsstand as on university library shelves. Population trends, data analysis techniques, and data sources are presented in a relevant and understandable manner. Health and fitness statistics and trend data are among the myriad subjects covered. However, because resources dealing solely with fitness statistics are not readily available, this magazine has a contribution to make.

B-60.   Blue Cross and Blue Shield of Indiana. **Health Promotion Service Evaluation and Impact Study**. Indianapolis, IN: Benchmark, 1986.

This study provides experimental data that demonstrate the cost-savings benefit for organizations if they will sponsor employee wellness programs. In 1977 Blue Cross and Blue Shield of Indiana (BCBSI) adopted a new health promotion program based on a model developed by the American Health Foundation. The BCBSI program focus shifted from illness treatment to health education. Efforts were oriented toward detecting and reducing health risk factors, absenteeism, and health care utilization costs. After five years, "reduced absenteeism and reduced utilization resulted in a return on investment of 2.51 to 1" (foreword). This study is well known because it provides proof that wellness programs are cost-effective. Other interested organizations can use it as a model to launch their own programs.

B-61.   Kelly, John R. **Recreation Business**. New York: Wiley, 1985.

This book aims to bring together the fields of business and recreation to introduce the concept of recreation business. Marketing and programming for recreation businesses are dependent on a knowledge of leisure participation patterns and demographic data on the target populations. Resources for obtaining needed market data are reviewed, basic economic definitions and concepts are reviewed, trends are extrapolated from available data, and vocational and business opportunities are suggested. For the convenience of the reader, chapter objectives are specified, issues are summarized, discussion questions are given, and possible projects are suggested. For those concerned with fitness and sports businesses, there are case studies of such businesses.

B-62.   **Nationwide Recreation Survey**. Washington, DC: National Park Service, 197?- . Irregular.

The responses of 5,757 Americans to the NRS provided information on their outdoor recreation activities – past, present, and future. For the first time, recreation behavior was surveyed by a consortium of federal agencies, resulting in a more comprehensive database than would otherwise have been possible. A computer tape of the NRS database, with documentation, is also available. Data were collected pertaining to: participation trends, favorite activities, preferred locations, use of national parks, trends in time/money expenditures, and activity patterns for senior citizens. Summary sections follow each chapter. Tables and figures explicate every aspect of the data collected. Fitness planners, promoters, and participants will find the survey useful to project trends across the total fitness industry.

Newsletters

B-63.   **Body Bulletin**. Emmaus, PA: Rodale, 1981- . Monthly.

Quick and easy health hints for mind and body are found in this newsletter. Articles and features are brief. Readers can find everything from capsule research reviews to recipes.

B-64. **Employee Health and Fitness**. Atlanta, GA: American Health Consultants, 1978- . Monthly.

Backed by an impressive advisory board composed of athletes, doctors, fitness consultants, executives, and educators, this is a substantial publication in terms of quantity and quality. The newsletter is advertised as "The executive update on health improvement programs," and its most appropriate audience would be those responsible for health care/wellness programs in an organization. Each issue discusses a topic in depth such as weight loss or managed care. The "Health and Well-Being" supplement appeals to the more general reader as well, because it contains books reviews, research findings, product reviews, and other news excerpted from a variety of sources. The cost may limit its circulation to larger libraries, health care organizations, and corporations that must keep current in this area.

B-65. **Executive Edge**. Emmaus, PA: Rodale, 1982- . Monthly.

The title is misleading because this newsletter should appeal to anyone with an interest in being effective, healthy, and happy on the job and at home. Content coverage ranges from managing stress to managing money. Features include book reviews, news, business trends, health hints, style and fashion updates, fitness tips, business travel do's and don'ts, and communication briefs. Both reasonably priced and successful in its mission to provide "useful information," this is a publication for a wide audience in a variety of work or home settings.

B-66. **Harvard Medical School Health Letter**. Boston: Department of Continuing Education, Harvard Medical School, 1975- . Monthly.

Designed to interpret medical information for the general reader, this newsletter discusses a limited number of topics per issue in some depth. Articles are not signed, but the editors and advisory board members are Harvard doctors. The content supports the preventive approach to health treatment and encourages the reader to participate in the health care process. This is a nonprofit newsletter, so it is affordable as well as informative.

B-67. **Running and FitNews**. Bethesda, MD: American Running and Fitness Association. 1984- . Monthly.

This is an example of a newsletter aimed at those who participate in a specific fitness activity. The association sponsoring it is composed of athletes and sports-medicine professionals. Articles often summarize research results and information from other cited sources. Some articles are signed. The editorial board includes such fitness experts as Kenneth Cooper, founder of the Aerobics Institute, and George Sheehan, cardiologist and author. "The Clinic" feature gives medical and training advice to readers who have requested information. This is a good awareness tool for the serious amateur or professional runner.

NOTES

[1]Claude Bouchard et al., *Exercise, Fitness and Health* (Champaign, IL: Human Kinetics, 1990), 6.

[2]Carl V. Gisolfi and David R. Lamb, *Youth Exercise and Sport* (Indianapolis, IN: Benchmark, 1989), 3.

[3]Ibid., 4.

[4]Ibid.

[5]Barry Glassner, "Fitness and the Postmodern Self," *Journal of Health and Social Behavior* 30 (1989): 180-91.

[6]Bouchard et al., 7.

[7]Ibid.

[8]Ardy Friedberg, *Facts on File Dictionary of Fitness* (New York: Facts on File, 1984), vii.

[9]Kenneth H. Cooper, *Aerobics* (New York: Bantam, 1968).

[10]James F. Fixx, *The Complete Book of Running* (New York: Random House, 1977).

[11]Friedberg, vii.

[12]James M. Rippe, *Dr. James M. Rippe's Fit for Success* (New York: Prentice-Hall, 1989), 34.

[13]Clayre K. Petray and Peter A. Cortese, "Physical Fitness: A Vital Component of the School Health Education Curriculum," *Health Education*, 19:5 (1988): 4-7.

[14]Petray and Cortese, 7.

[15]Lawrence W. Green and Frances M. Lewis, *Measurement and Evaluation in Health Education and Health Promotion* (Palo Alto, CA: Mayfield, 1986), xvii.

[16]David H. Chenoweth, *Planning Health Promotion at the Worksite* (Indianapolis, IN: Benchmark, 1987), 9.

[17]Dale Feuer, "Wellness Programs," *Training*, 22:4 (1985): 25-34.

[18]Bud Getchell, *The Fitness Book* (Indianapolis, IN: Benchmark, 1987), 3.

[19]Bouchard et al., 7.

[20]Robert K. Cooper, *Health and Fitness Excellence* (Boston: Houghton Mifflin, 1989), xii.

[21]Glassner, 180.

[22]Tom Fennell and D'arcy Jenish, "The Riches of Sport," *Macleans*, 103:15 (1990): 42-45.

[23]Ibid., 41.

[24]Feuer, 32.

[25]Blue Cross and Blue Shield of Indiana, *Health Promotion Service Evaluation and Impact Study* (Indianapolis, IN: Benchmark, 1986).

[26]Rippe, 52.

[27]*Stanford Health and Exercise Handbook* (Champaign, IL: Leisure Press, 1989), 183.

[28]"Good Sense, Good Health," *Sports Illustrated*, 13 November 1989, 15.

[29]Green and Lewis, xvii.

[30]Glassner, 180.

[31]Ibid., 187.

[32]Feuer, 30.

[33]Roy J. Shephard, *Economic Benefits of Enhanced Fitness* (Champaign, IL: Human Kinetics, 1986), 265.

[34]"The Recreation, Fitness and Leisure Industry in 1988," *Recreation, Sports and Leisure* (July/August 1988): 5-6, 8-9, 12-13.

[35]Feuer, 25.

[36]Glassner, 183.

[37]Ibid., 182.

[38]Peri Caylor, "Fitness 1990," *American Fitness* (January/February 1990): 20-22.

[39]Green and Lewis, 3.

[40]Chenoweth, 10.

[41]Marjory Roberts and T. George Harris, "Wellness at Work," *Psychology Today* 23 (1989): 54-58.

[42]Janette Scandura, "Beefing Up a Skinny Business," *Working Woman*, February 1990, 53-58.

[43]Joseph Kotarba and Pamela Bentley, "Workplace Wellness Participation and the Becoming of Self," *Social Science and Medicine*, 26:5 (1988): 551-58.

[44]Patricia Braus, "A Workout for the Bottom Line," *American Demographics*, 11:10 (1989): 34-37, 59.

[45]Feuer, 32.

[46]Green and Lewis, 24.

[47]Blue Cross and Blue Shield, x.

[48]Feuer, 32.

[49]Green and Lewis, 3.

[50]Rippe, 26.

[51]John D. Adams, "A Healthy Cut in Costs," *Personnel Administrator*, 33 (August 1988): 42-47.

[52]Caylor, 22.

[53]Green and Lewis, xi.

[54]Ibid.

[55]Robert Cooper, ix.

[56]Gisolfi and Lamb, xi.

[57]Joseph P. Opatz, ed., *Wellness Promotion Strategies* (Stevens Point, WI: University of Wisconsin, 1984).

[58]*Stanford Health and Exercise Handbook*, 33.

[59]Ibid., 34.

[60]Carol Krucoff, "Has Fitness Fizzled?" *The Washington Post*, 3 January 1990, 27.

[61]Roberts and Harris, 54-56, 58.

[62]Rippe, 27.

[63]John R. Kelly, "Recreation Trends," *Business* 38 [formerly *Atlanta Economic Review*] (April, May, June 1988): 54-57.

[64]Feuer, 28.

[65]Glassner, 184.

[66]Chenoweth, 200-206.

[67]AAHPERD, *Physical Education Gold Book* (Champaign, IL: Human Kinetics, 1987), 1-33.

[68]See the *Peterson's Guide to Four-Year Colleges, Peterson's Guide to Graduate Programs in Business, Education, Health and Law* (Princeton, NJ: Peterson's Guides, 1989); *Graduate Program Directory* (Indianapolis, IN: ASCM, 1990); and *Annual Information Directory* (Stamford, CT: Association for Fitness in Business, 1988).

[69]Program descriptions taken from *Peterson's Guide to Graduate Programs in Business, Education, Health and Law*.

[70]Chenoweth, 204-6.

[71]Bouchard, 31.

[72]John Naisbitt and Patricia Aburdene, *Megatrends 2000* (New York: Morrow, 1990).

[73]Nancy Giges, "Health Trend Hits Life-Style Mainstream," *Advertising Age*, 17 February 1986, 58.

[74]Glassner, 183.

[75]Ibid.

[76]Giges, 58.

[77]Ibid.

[78]Kotarba and Bentley, 558.

[79]Kelly, 56.

[80]Caylor, 22.

[81]Marilu D. Meredith, "Activity or Fitness: Is the Process or the Product More Important for Public Health?" *Quest*, 40 (1980): 180-86.

[82]Judith Waldrop, "Feeling Good," *American Demographics*, May 1989, 6.

[83]Roy J. Shephard, *Fitness in Special Populations* (Champaign, IL: Human Kinetics, 1990), viii.

[84]Ibid., 229.

[85]*National Recreation Survey* (Washington, DC: National Park Service, 1982-83), 5.

[86]*Philadelphia Inquirer*, 13 September 1990, 7-WHF.

[87]Barbara A. Johnson, "A Community Walks for Wellness," *Journal of Physical Education, Recreation and Dance*, 59 (1988): 64-67.

[88]Ellen Kunes, "No Sweat Fitness," *Working Woman*, April 1990, 119-20.

[89]Bob Glover and Jack Shepard, *The Family Fitness Handbook* (New York: Penguin, 1989), 335.

[90]Chenoweth, 9.

[91]Braus, 37.

[92]Feuer, 30.

[93]Ibid., 25.

[94]Caylor, 22.

THE LITERATURE OF SPORT

Mila C. Su

INTRODUCTION

What exactly is sport? It is not simply the participation in athletic games for fun and recreation. For example, the term *sport* is also applied to the hunting of wild animals, to game fishing, and to betting on horse and dog races. "From the simple notion of sport as an amusement, we come down to the curiously specialized uses of the word which tie it down on the one hand to pursuits of killing and on the other to games in which a money stake is involved."[1] Sport is an ambiguous term that has no standard definition. Generally, it is agreed that sports are competitive and formalized games requiring physical skills. However, even those who study and write about sport have not developed a uniform definition.

Sport is also distinct from the related activities of play, games, and athletics. Play is first associated with childhood, with situations that are made up, changed at whim, and played as long as they are fun. "Play" has an even broader meaning than "sport" or "games," encompassing "any activity that is free, separate, uncertain, spontaneous, unproductive, and governed by rules and make-believe."[2]

In contrast, games can be fun but might require more organization than play; they are one form of playful competition in which the outcome is determined by physical skill, strategy, or chance—employed singly or in combination.[3] According to John W. Loy, games are considered friendly and/or recreational until they reach tournament level; then they become sport.[4] Paul Weiss suggests that when the term "game" is interchanged with the term "sport," it implies "idle conformity to rules"[5] and that games are usually pursued for fun even though there is a winner, a loser, and some sort of physical or mental strategy.

Athletics are marked by intense competition. An athlete is an individual who has acquired certain great physical strengths through special training and exercise. The term *athletics* is defined as a contest with prizes where winners demonstrate their superiority. Harold J. VanderZwaag describes an athlete as one who is driven by the pursuit of excellence.[6] Society, however, perceives the athlete as one motivated primarily by the desire to win.

One current taxonomy of sport, made by Stephen K. Figler, begins with play as the most general development, then games, then sports, and then the most specific form—athletics.[7] He defines play as "activity that tends not to be limited in time and space."[8] In contests, games have limitations in space and time and include the understanding that ultimately there will be a winner and a loser. "This is a key distinction between games and play.... In other words, games are primarily recreational, with relaxation, exercise, human interaction, and enjoyment providing the primary motivations."[9] He continues, "sports are significantly more competitive than games, and it follows that there is significantly more investment of time, energy, money, and ego in sports ... and concern for won-lost records."[10] This author portrays athletics as being more serious than sports: "Sports are basically pleasurable diversions characterized by moderate effort, while participation in athletics is characterized by intense dedication and sacrifice."[11]

Athletics are also performed on a variety of levels. An amateur athlete is considered to be one who does not make a professional living in a particular sporting contest. Currently, the determination of amateur status is very controversial, especially in Olympics and collegiate level competition. Amateur competitions include but are not limited to the Olympics, the Junior Olympics, the Pan-American Games, and the World Games. The terms *college athletics* or *intercollegiate athletics* are used to refer to varsity sports in any division. *Intramural clubs* are defined as team and individual sports that allow students within an institution to participate and compete against one another. *Extramural clubs* are individual and team sports that receive some financial support from the parent institution and that function in compliance with established club rules and regulations. These clubs have divisions similar to those of intercollegiate teams and competition within their divisions is just as fierce.

High school or interscholastic sports also have several competitive levels within four divisions: AAAA, AAA, AA, and A. Park and recreation activities also overlap with sport. They are usually outdoor activities controlled by the state or local park service. But persons who participate in sports in an informal sense—that is, for pleasure and enjoyment during their free time—are considered in the literature to be *recreating*. Recreation is a very general term, which applies to participating in any and all leisure activity.

INTERDISCIPLINARY NATURE OF SPORT

To study sport one must examine a wide variety of fields that fall into two basic categories:

1. The sport sciences (treatment and prevention of injuries and the enhancement of performance). These include biomechanics, kinesiology, exercise physiology, sports medicine, sports psychology, motor learning, and ergometrics.

2. The social sciences (theoretical examination of the social aspects of sport). These include areas like the history of sport, the philosophy in and of sport, the psychology of sport, and the sociology of sport.

HISTORY OF SPORT

The history of sport in America has been examined by historians, sociologists, and philosophers because sport has traditionally been viewed by them as a microcosm of the society in which they live. Research shows that native Americans used sport as a ceremonial or ritual activity to express attitudes and values. Native American cultures valued physical prowess, so games and sport had an important role in daily and holiday activities. When the pilgrims and other European settlers came to North America they not only brought their games and sports from their homelands, they also brought their attitudes and beliefs toward the place of sport in society. Their religion, however, had an important influence on sport and usually tried to restrict the amount of play in its members' free time. Some churches opposed leisurely pursuits and attacked sport as sinful.[12] But colleges and universities in colonial America were based on English academic institutional models, and soon after their establishment, students aggressively petitioned for the formal inclusion of sports into academic life. The first intercollegiate competition, a crew meet between Harvard and Yale, was recorded in 1852. This marked the first step in the gradual evolution of competitive American sport. "Intercollegiate sport, after that first meet, grew up with the emergence of industrial America. Colleges and their sports took on many of the features of the larger America and its capitalistic rush for wealth, power, recognition, and influence."[13] Religious pressure for limiting sport participation was fading.

On the frontier, life involved sporting contests such as plowing contests and logging competitions that developed in conjunction with work. In the cities, urban dwellers were affected by the industrial revolution. It is well documented that during the mid-1800s the rise of sport for the general populace began. Competition developed in such sports as tennis and bicycling for both sexes and over time these sports increased in popularity.[14] Athletic clubs grew in abundance too. The number of clubs made possible a new mission—training for competition in track and field events. In fact, Americans, borrowing from their ancestors, took the European definition of "athletics" to mean track and field. Nothing, not even the outbreak of the Civil War, impeded citizens from actively pursuing the sporting life.

Sports events such as baseball, prize fighting, and horse racing were transported to different regions of the country with the advent of the railroad and the resulting western expansion. In 1869, the first professional baseball team was formed. About the same time, park and recreation activities sprung up in communities across America, and by 1896 the modern international Olympics were initiated. Locally, service and recreational programs provided outlets for growing boys. Organized youth agencies in America started in 1851 with the establishment of the Young Men's Christian Association (YMCA) in Boston and the Boy Scouts of America.[15] These programs were intended to mold young men into well-rounded citizens and to keep them out of trouble. As the century progressed, in both rural and urban settings, churches lost their previous fear of sport and free time and began developing active sports programs: "To meet the social needs of rural and city members, churches adopted sports and sponsored recreation to draw people together, and church leadership played an important role in the promotion of community recreation."[16]

Leisure time became a reality for the masses when the industrial revolution prompted legislative changes in the work routine, especially the limiting of the number of hours in the work week. With workers protected from abuses by factory owners and children regaining their time to play, an increase in sports activity was natural. Growing inner cities and expanding suburbs were identified as places that needed to offer play areas for youth and adults. Between World War I and World War II, sport became an acceptable vehicle of education. But as the programs expanded and grew, problems began to develop. Difficulties in collegiate football such as dirty play, cheating, and illegal gambling led to the organization of the Intercollegiate Athletic Association of the United States (IAA) in 1905. The formation of the National Collegiate Athletic Association (NCAA) quickly followed. "The IAA began to clean up football, particularly its brutality. In 1910 this organization became the NCAA and expanded its mission to cover all unethical conduct in collegiate athletics."[17] The installation of the IAA and the permanent establishment of the NCAA was the beginning of organizations in sport that manage, oversee, and enforce rules, regulations, and guidelines. Formally organized youth sport was established separately from the educational system. For example, the Pop Warner Leagues were established in 1929 and ten years later Little League play was in full swing. "New organizations for boys came into existence as separate enterprises. They were recreational rather than evangelical in nature, primarily because the character building values were thought to be interrelated to play, games, and sport."[18]

ECONOMICS

Economics played an important part in the status and structure of sport. New technology in communicating information was quickly adapted and incorporated to relay sport information. In the 1900s newspapers reported sport scores and sport information, and by the 1920s, radio was broadcasting sporting events such as baseball, football, and boxing in a play-by-play format. The innovation of the electric light also had enormous impact on sport, allowing indoor and outdoor sport participation anytime, day or night. "Within a few years electric lighting and more comfortable accommodations helped lure players and spectators alike to YMCA's athletic clubs, regimental armories, school and college gymnasiums, as well as sports arenas."[19]

Radio, which survived the Depression, entertained Americans during World War II and "never before had entertainment become not only such a big business in itself, but also an integral part of the country's basic economic system."[20]

Following World War II, a new sense of economics and leisure developed. Families not only were more prosperous, but they also had more free time.

More money bought state-of-the-art technology and technology brought sport into the home. The shift from radio to television happened rapidly during the 1950s and caused citizens to withdraw from the public arena to the security of their own homes. "In the post-World War II era, there was a shift from inner-city, public forms for recreation to private, home-centered forms of recreation."[21] Television technology would continue to influence sport for decades. Not only were networks, leagues, and teams created to generate money, but spectators were allowed the luxury of watching at home. "Almost single-handedly the new electronic medium revolutionized the economics of big-time sport ... soaring television revenues helped induce numerous franchise shifts and a rapid increase in the number of professional sport franchises."[22] The media received the protection of the copyright law with the passing of the Media Copyright Act of 1976, which gave sports organizations a right to copyright the broadcasts of their games or contests.[23]

Acting as an external force, television

> performs this pivotal role primarily by creating, promoting, and organizing highly lucrative sports markets. Professional sports were not the only ones affected by the seduction of media revenues and publicity; college athletics also jumped on the television band-wagon. Television occupies this niche in corporate athleticism because it has the ability to organize mass appeal.[24]

Nand Hart-Nibbring considers "corporate athleticism" to be the commercialization of college sports in which amateur athletes mimic the expectations that the professional sports have concerning money, winning, and status.[25]

POLITICS

Sport has a political dimension as well. The president of the United States puts an investment in the youth and adults of America through the President's Council on Physical Fitness and Sports. Even the Olympics has been politicized. "Sport always has been seen as a visible and effective means to communicate national and international policy."[26] Money and favoritism go to schools, sports, and individuals because of successful sports participation. And political and legislative intervention and interference legitimize sport as an investment.

Sport is perceived by businesses and communities as a revenue-producing venture, and they have lobbied for policies to protect their investment. "Amateur and professional sports are items on the agendas of various public policy-making institutions, and sports activities are affected in myriad ways by public policy decisions.[27] As with any other business, the development of sport into big business has required government intervention to ensure that monopolies and discrimination do not occur. "Sport has acquired the status of a *public trust*, which must be protected. As a result, public policy in the form of law or regulatory action has been implemented to guarantee the public equitable access."[28] Government intervention can be a two-edged sword. A sense of nationalism and regionalism are often found in identifying with a particular team. "Sport also can promote a feeling of community attachment and goodwill among citizens, as well as provide the impetus for surges of patriotism and national pride in general."[29]

In contrast, when the government interceded for political reasons in the 1980 Olympic boycott, many athletes expressed their dissatisfaction with this decision. Issues of racial and gender discrimination are also often tied to politics. Legislators have helped fight for more equality in sport by providing legal grounds to strengthen plaintiffs' cases. When the civil rights legislation was extended to African-Americans, it also protected other minority groups against incidents of discrimination. As a result, many have argued that sport is an area where there is more equality than in the larger society. However, several authors have pointed out the tendency of African-Americans and other minorities to occupy "certain positions" in certain sports while the whites on the team play more of the "glory" positions. Figler comments:

> While physiological differences may partially explain the prevalence of blacks in some sports and at some positions, ... a fuller explanation comes from inclusion of such sociology factors as geography, ... access to coaching, economics, lack of social mobility opportunities in some sports, as well as "good old, down home" biogotry. But the most heavily emphasized reason offered by sociologists seems to be the absence of black role models along with the absence of money-making opportunities in these other sports.[30]

There are several ways a player can file his or her grievance, depending on the grievance and the level of athletics. "Athletes are becoming aware of their rights today, not only under the Fourteenth Amendment but also under the First, Fourth, Fifth and Ninth."[31]

WOMEN'S ROLE IN SPORT

In 1972 Title IX of the Education Amendment gave females a legal means to fight for their rights to participate and receive support in sports. Institutions were given until 1978 to implement programs for girls and women that were comparable to male programs. There were many court cases during this time — including the landmark case of Grove City College vs. Bell — as schools, colleges, and even the NCAA fought against this legislation. Women's organizations such as SPRINT[32] and the Association of Intercollegiate Athletics for Women (AIAW) were established to help support females in sport. The AIAW represented women in athletics and fought against the NCAA to have provisions included for women athletes. In 1981 when the NCAA finally agreed to change its policies to reflect equal access for both sexes, it merged with the AIAW. Unfortunately, this incorporation has eliminated the functions of the AIAW.

As female teams achieve great success, coaches find they need to recruit just as heavily as for their male counterparts. However, there are still inequalities, which have forced many teams to look to corporate sponsors. There also have been more sponsors willing to support sports for women, including golf, tennis, basketball, softball, and volleyball. One of the controversies that has arisen out of this competitive recruiting is over the fact that women's sport is turning out to be a copy of the men's.

> Title IX provides for rapid and immediate expansion, leaving behind concern for well-considered direction. In our zeal to avoid subjecting women to more discrimination, we seem to be fostering the development of the same faulty mechanism that drives men's school athletic programs.[33]

Only time will tell which direction women's sports will follow.

LAW

Another legal development that protected athletes from ethnic and gender discrimination was the Amateur Sports Act passed by Congress in 1978. The act reorganized and coordinated amateur athletics in the United States. Its mission was to encourage and strengthen participation of U.S. amateurs in international competition. The United States Olympic Committee (USOC) was established as the principal mechanism for attaining these objectives. "It creates a governing structure for the USOC by empowering it to select one National Governing Body for each Olympic or Pan-American sport."[34] The act concerns itself primarily with the relationship between athletes eligible for international amateur competition and the ruling bodies that govern those competitions as well as relationships among the ruling bodies themselves.

A clause within the Amateur Act ensures that all handicapped persons will have equal opportunities to participate in athletic programs.[35] It also provides special athletic opportunities for those unable to participate in regular athletic programs.[36] The distinction between handicapped and disabled is that *handicapped* refers to a barrier—physical, emotional, or mental—that keeps one from reaching his or her goals; *disabled* refers to a condition that is clinically describable. According to Claudine Sherrell, the term "handicapped" generally refers to children in school while "disabled" is used for adults and athletes. Disabled athletes fall into the following categories: amputee, blind, cerebral palsy, spinal cord injured, and *les autres*. Each category has a range of classifications, which enable each athlete to be assessed with athletes of equal abilities. There are a variety of associations that sponsor competitions for these individuals such as the Paraolympics, which was held in Seoul in 1984. The special Olympian, unlike the previously mentioned disabled athletes, is mentally retarded. Many are multidisabled with a combination of mental, physical, or emotional disabilities.[37]

The creation of these laws required lawyers to move into the realm of sport. Sports law focuses heavily on the area of injury, which is governed by tort law. Other litigation has related to the failure or improper fit of equipment and the failure to maintain facilities. Within the last five years an increasing number of spectators have sued clubs, players, and facilities for injuries they have sustained. "The United States is becoming a nation of spectators as evidenced by the record breaking crowds at almost every type of sports event. It seems logical that increased attendance will lead to situations that result in litigation."[38]

Legal statutes and precedents have affected sport in new ways. "On a general level, the cases in the mid-70's served to finally strip away the myth that sports activities were recreational in nature and, thus not subject to close scrutiny."[39] Government will continue to intercede with laws and regulations or rules in specific cases. "The sports industry therefore has become a legitimate area of interest for government, and sports policy is evolving into a distinct policy area analogous to housing, energy, public health, and other commonly recognized fields. As a result, government is asked to do more than settle internecine disputes within the sports industry."[40]

ETHICS IN SPORT

A hot topic in the literature of sports recently has been the issue of ethics. Ethics in sport encompass the philosophy of fair and foul play as well as how the players, spectators, media, and society in general influence its perception. Ethics are often associated with the public's perception of the sports world and its many related elements: the fading of the amateur athlete concept, violence, drugs, gender and race issues, injuries, the "winning at all costs" theory, gambling, and the marketing and business aspects of sport.

America's view of sport has changed in the past twenty years, and present attitudes often lose sight of its original goals, which were to develop attitudes of strength of character and fair play. A winning performance versus sportsman-like conduct is one conflict often debated now in articles and editorials; amateur/professional status for Olympians is another; and the issue of academic standards for collegiate athletes has created numerous citations as has that of drugs and sports. During the next decade these and many more issues will be studied from historical, sociological, psychological, and medical perspectives in the literature of sport.

ACADEMICS

The study of sport has three basic thrusts: (1) sports study with an educational emphasis; (2) sports study with a scientific emphasis; and (3) sports study with a broader social science emphasis. "Sport is one of the most pervasive social phenomena of the Twentieth Century. Not only is it a popular leisure activity, but a social institution that permeates several aspects of social life."[41] Sport study has become a part of most postsecondary institutions' curricula and has expanded to the master's and doctoral levels of study in large universities in the United States, Canada, and the United Kingdom. The study of sport can be divided into three major fields: physical education, sport sciences, and the sociology of sport.

The most traditional avenue to the study of sport has been through its educational affiliation, the study of physical education. Physical education is defined as the training and teaching of individuals to develop a sense of their own physical being. It has been incorporated into the structure of elementary and high school environments and has required certified professionals to teach it as a subject. "By its very title, physical education is physical activity with an educational goal. It is physical and it seeks to educate, but neither play nor sport — even though both can be used in the educational process — always includes the educational portion of the physical experience as a vital aim."[42]

Physical education has not been taken very seriously by academicians in the past. Much of the sport and athletic activity in past academic programs was administered by the physical education department, and there continues to be very little distinction made by society and the academic community between teaching classes in physical education and coaching competitive sports. "Many physical education educators have wanted to divorce themselves from this tie to sports in the belief that only in this way can physical education show its true worth in the educational arenas."[43] The common misunderstanding of physical education is the failure to make this distinction and the failure to understand the importance of proper education in health and physical being. At the college, university, and high school levels, physical education courses are offered, and students are required to earn a number of such credits in order to graduate. These courses are sometimes identified as contributing to the confusion in the physical education discipline today.

Sports science moves the study of sport out of the general education arena into the world of the hard sciences, the medical sciences, and the health sciences. Emphasis is placed on quantifiable measurement, on hypotheses, and on research and development. Sports science can be studied at undergraduate, master's and doctoral levels. It includes physiology, kinesiology, motor learning, biomechanics, and medicine. Biomechanics, locomotion studies, and motor skill programs have found athletes to be wonderful subjects for the study of specific conditions that can be manipulated and imitated.

The academic study of sports can also be traced through its ties to sociology and antecedents in such social sciences as anthropology, history, psychology, and geography. Academic programs for this type of study are becoming extremely popular at undergraduate and graduate levels. Social sport study usually includes courses in psychology, administration of sport, sociology, philosophy, and history. By the 1980s study in sport law also developed into a speciality. And sport media has subcategories such as journalism (newspapers and magazines) and communications (radio, TV, video, filming, and photography). Related educational programs in sport include those for rehabilitation, physical therapy, athletic trainers, facilities maintenance, turf maintenance, and sport information directors (who deal with statistics and public relations information).

Fields that are cross-disciplinary with and related to sport include geography/demographics, women's studies, economics, business, and marketing. The expansion of the sport concept into the business arena has been meteoric but at a price. "As sport has become increasingly 'worklike' and professionalized, the concepts and the methods used to analyze sport have become similar to those in any other industry."[44]

With the swing in social attitudes toward sport and sports activities, there is an opportunity for more universal acceptance of academic learning across age groups. Lifelong learning skills, corporate fitness, and adaptive physical education are just a few of the current growing areas in sport education that can be expanded on many academic levels. The fields of formal sport study are still evolving. Professionals in these areas have discussed the need to show that sport study is as rigorous as other academic concentrations.

PRODUCERS OF DATA

The chief producers of sports information are: (1) private companies (including the sporting goods industry and the insurance industry); (2) research and academic centers; (3) professional athletic associations; and (4) governmental agencies at all levels. Data from these four areas relate to any specific sport, sport trends, sport problems, or any area that is identified as having information of interest to the field of sport science. Data are gathered through every possible research method but the most popular methods include interviews, experiments, and surveys. Observation is also frequently employed.

Sports workers today are gravitating to the business and economic sides of the industry, frequently allying themselves with the entertainment industry for operational models for managing a team, issuing contracts, handling players, dealing with agents, satisfying unions, managing public relations, and managing the facilities that house sporting events. All of these activities require the support of an ever-expanding literature of sport that provides access to information needed for successful sports management and administration.

Two important industries contribute to the literature of sport. The sporting goods industry plays a part in the corporate sponsorship of amateur, college, and professional events, teams, and individuals. Like the sporting goods industry, the sports insurance industry is a multifaceted one that plays an important role in the economics of sport and contributes a large body of information to the field. Individuals, teams, facilities, spectators, and special events all need to have insurance coverage to protect against litigation. Insurance companies gather data concerning specific sports and specific sport-related injuries. The *Insurance Periodical Index* is invaluable in locating information on topics related to sports injuries and sports medicine lawsuits and claims.

Marketing, advertising, and communications operations are also very important contributors to the literature of sport. Television, cable networks, videos, radio stations, magazines, newspapers, and books all disseminate information about sports around the world daily. Athletes who are rated as role models or as heroes have marketing values assigned to them and are regularly hired for product endorsements.

Often private companies such as American Sports Data Incorporated and Sports Research Incorporated collect, produce, manipulate, and sell sports data. These data are tailored to meet the needs of individual clients. Companies spend considerable time and effort to collect information, which makes data collection expensive. The information is not considered to be in the public domain and it is not usually disclosed or made accessible to the general public. These companies can be located through directories such as the *Sport Market Place* or through journals such as *Athletic Business*.

Sport research centers such as the Sport Information Resource Centre can be independent or they can be affiliated with academic institutions such as the centers located at Arizona State University and the University of Southern California. These centers focus on a range of sport issues, although the majority concentrate on issues relating to sports medicine and injuries. The knowledge produced by these centers is incorporated with other aspects of sport science in order to improve athletic performance. Academic research centers tend to specialize in sport sciences. Some examples include Temple University's Center for Sports Medicine and Science, the University of Denver's Sport Science Lab, and Pennsylvania State University's Locomotion Laboratory. They can be independent centers, laboratories, or laboratories in classrooms where upper-level undergraduates and graduate students observe the biomechanics of an individual's movements, motor skills, locomotion, and improvements in sports performance. These laboratories also study related issues such as aging and disease (diabetes, asthma, etc.) and their impact on both athletes and nonathletes. Other academic centers such as the North-western Center for the Study of Sport focus on the social aspects of sport. Some research centers make their data available through local databases such as the Leisure Studies Data Base, produced by the University of Waterloo and the United States Olympic Center.

The following professional associations play a major role in the development and distribution of sports-related data: the Sporting Goods Association, the American Alliance for Health, Physical Education, Recreation and Dance, and the Women's Sport Foundation. These groups not only gather data but they also conduct studies of primary concern to their members. The types of publications they produce include directories, periodicals, annual reports, newsletters, and conference proceedings.

Athletic organizations such as the United States Olympic Committee, the National Governing Bodies, National Collegiate Athletic Association, National Junior Collegiate Athletic Association, and the National Association for Intercollegiate Athletics produce academic institution records such as win/loss records, player awards, and rules violations statistics. This information is available in their publications.

Government agencies at all levels produce information on sports. Data relating to injuries, sports industries, demographics, education, and many other issues may be accessed through statistical indexes such as the *American Statistical Index* and the *Statistical Reference Index*.

RESEARCH

Sport research has identified problems, defined areas needing further study, has led to improvements in individual performance, and has contributed to the creation of new and better products for use in athletic competition. Research methodologies range from field work and observation to the analysis and use of secondary data sources. Sports research is generally classified into one of two areas: (1) sport sciences or the social aspects of sport and (2) sport science research, which has four basic areas of study—improvement in health and physical performance, injury prevention, equipment design, and improvement of athletic performance.

All of the resources that follow in this chapter have been selected to provide fast, easy-to-use, current information in the field of sport and sport-related subject areas.

SOURCES

Guides and Handbooks

C-1. Goldberger, Alan S. **Sports Officiating: A Legal Guide**. Westpoint, NY: Leisure Press, 1984.
This monograph provides insight into the legal obligations of officiating. It is a good introduction to the subject and serves as a checklist of legal issues related to officiating. Chapters cover pregame duties, lawsuits, individual sports (baseball, basketball, football, soccer, and wrestling), postgame activities, and injury situations. There are also descriptions of official associations. Appendices include a discussion of overall responsibility in interscholastic sport ranging from the board of directors to pep clubs. A subject index is included.

C-2. Gratch, Bonnie, comp. **Sports and Physical Education: A Guide to Reference Resources**. Westport, CT: Greenwood Press, 1983.
This guide is divided into three parts: (1) individual sports, based on Ralph Hickok's chapter on the Olympics in *New Encyclopedia of Sports* (entry C-33); (2) sports and physical education (general and topical); and (3) indexes, databases, and information centers. Access is enhanced by author (personal and corporate), title, and subject indexes. The 624 entries have brief but informative annotations to various reference resources in physical education, sports, and allied fields. The resources consist of English-language materials published in the United States, Canada, and the United Kingdom for 1970-82.

C-3. Higgs, Robert J. **Sports: A Reference Guide**. Westport, CT: Greenwood Press, 1982.
The topics covered in the fourteen chapters range from a history of sports to traditional arts and sports. Also included are other important topics rarely discussed in the literature such as sport and its relation to popular culture, education, money and social values, race, sex, fans, and aggression. There is a brief American chronology and a list of research centers in the appendices. Each chapter contains an essay consisting of comments and notations of references relevant to the subject matter and a nonannotated bibliography. Journal articles and books are included in the bibliography. There are two appendices: a chronology of American sport and a list of various research centers, collections, and directories.

C-4. Killpatrick, Frances, and James Killpatrick. **The Winning Edge: A Complete Guide to Athletic Programs**. Chicago: Longman, 1989.
This book is the most complete guide to scholarships and sources of financial assistance in sports. It details rules and regulations governing financial aid. It provides college program descriptions of various sports. For each school there are summary tables for the following data: school name; telephone number; participation in national

and regional conferences; annual budget information; and lists of physical education programs including baseball, basketball, crewing, fencing, field hockey, football, golf, gymnastics, ice hockey, lacrosse, skiing, soccer, squash, swimming, tennis, track, volleyball, and wrestling. Sports are classified as men's or women's and levels of competitiveness are indicated. Program descriptions also provide information on budgets and staffing (coaches and assistant coaches), full and partial scholarships, conference winnings, pro drafts and seating capacity in sports facilities for football, basketball, and ice hockey. There is even a list for club sports for both sexes.

C-5.   Loy, John W., Barry D. McPherson, and Gerald Kenyon. **Sport and Social Systems: A Guide to the Analysis, Problems and Literature**. Reading, MA: Addison-Wesley, 1978.

Loy and his coauthors Barry McPherson and Gerald Kenyon are familiar names in the literature of the social aspects of sport. This resource provides excellent insight into and background on all components and related areas of the sociology of sport. Many issues of concern today are highlighted, including the special phenomena of sport, the micro/macro levels of sport, and the institution of sport. Each chapter includes a list of suggested additional references.

C-6.   Prytherch, Ray. **Sports and Fitness: An Information Guide**. Brookfield, VT: Gower, 1988.

This work presents sport information from a librarian's perspective but is also useful for other researchers involved in exploring professional and/or amateur sport. Although emphasizing British sports, it provides a solid model for sports research in any country. It explores research techniques in sport sciences and discusses statistical analyses used by special groups. Prytherch lists resources that fall between scholarly and general use materials and includes diagrams and examples of sport terminology. Indexes are provided.

C-7.   Remley, Mary L. **Women in Sport: A Guide to Information Sources**. Sports, Games and Pastimes Information Guide. 10 vol. Detroit: Gale Research Co., 1980.

This book provides over 300 annotated titles of general reference works, biographies, books on techniques and instruction, periodicals, films, and other sources for organizations/halls of fame. In addition to these categories, over fifty additional titles are recommended, including materials for youth/popular readings. A list of organizations is provided. There are author, title, and subject indexes.

C-8.   Remley, Mary L. **Women in Sport: An Annotated Bibliography and Resource Guide, 1900-1990**. Boston: G. K. Hall, 1991.

This publication, an updated version of the author's 1980 publication on *Women in Sport* (entry C-7), functions as a guide to the literature and a bibliographic resource all in one volume. It brings together publications on women in sports published since 1900. Its compiler, a professor of kinesiology and women's studies, arranged over 700 entries chronologically by year and alphabetically within each year. The first four chapters cover the following time frames: 1900-30, 1931-60, 1961-75, and 1976-90. A final chapter covers such entries as periodical titles that focus on women's sports. Author, title, and subject indexes complete this very useful and up-to-date volume.

C-9.   Salmela, John H. **The World Sport Psychology Sourcebook**. Ithaca, NY: Movement Publishers, 1981.

Salmela presents in this work a global listing and discussion of sport psychology programs arranged by country or geographical location. The book is divided into three sections: (1) basic questions and answers in sport psychology; (2) a world perspective of sport psychology; and (3) a *Who's Who* of sport psychology. An updated edition is expected in 1991-92.

Standard/Classic Sources

C-10.   Ashe, Arthur R. **A Hard Road to Glory: A History of the African American**. 3 vols. New York: Warner Books, 1988.

This work explores the history and development of the African-American athlete. The first volume covers 1619 to 1918; the second, 1919 to 1945; and the third, 1946 to 1988. The coverage is limited to the sports of baseball, basketball, tennis, and bowling. Each volume contains three sections: (1) an essay covering the historical background of the sport; (2) a reference section providing lists of players, school records, names of coaches, and other types of statistical information; and (3) a repeated bibliography in each volume divided into monograph and serial categories. A small list of organizations and foundations is also provided.

C-11.   Caillois, Roger. **Man, Play and Games**. Translated by Meyer Barash. New York: Free Press, 1961.

In this classic work Caillois goes several steps beyond John Huizinga's evaluation of play (entry C-13). He includes games and sports as part of its evolution and comments further on play, games, and sports' relationship to society. This book is one of the earliest comprehensive treatises analyzing the role of play, games, sport, and society.

C-12.   Dulles, Foster Rhea. **America Learns to Play: A History of Popular Recreation**. 2d ed. New York: Appleton-Century-Crofts, 1965.

Dulles follows the evolution of recreation and leisure's role in American society. From the history of the earliest settlers to the atmosphere of sport in the 1930s, the author explores how games, play, and eventually sport were perceived by the people of the times and how the changes influenced society. This outstanding work ties together the development of recreation and sport with the growth of American society. A bibliography is included.

C-13.   Huizinga, John. **Homo Ludens: A Study of the Play Element in Culture**. New York: Harper & Row, 1970.

Huizinga is credited with being the catalyst for the examination and study of play. This classic book is crucial to any discussion of the theory of play in which the activity is defined in historical and societal perspective.

C-14.   Lucas, John A., and Ronald A. Smith. **The Saga of Sport**. Philadelphia, PA: Lea & Lebiger, 1978.

This classic is one of the most often quoted resources in the literature of sport and offers a solid introduction to the history of sport in America. It is divided into three sections: (1) colonial and early America, the puritans to the Civil War; (2) American sport in transition, the development of the organization of sport; and (3) sport in the twentieth century, the emergence of professionalism in American sport, and issues of race and sex.

C-15. Sherrill, Claudine. **Adapted Physical Education and Recreation: A Multidisciplinary Approach**. 3d ed. Dubuque, IA: William C. Brown, 1986.

Sherrill provides a standard work covering every aspect of adapted physical education. The work is divided into three parts: (1) quality physical education for all students; (2) service delivery and individual education programs; and (3) adapted physical education. There are many chapters in each section as well as an extensive bibliography.

C-16. Tutko, Thomas. **Sport Psyching: Playing Your Best Game All of the Time**. New York: Hawthorne Books, 1976.

Tutko provides a well-written source that explains the fundamentals of sport psychology. The book is designed for individuals to easily evaluate and define their own psychological perceptions of sport. Dorcas S. Butt's *Psychology of Sport* and R. B. Alderman's *Psychological Behavior of Sport* are two other important books from this period that present a more academic perspective.

C-17. Weiss, Paul. **Sport: A Philosophic Inquiry**. Carbondale, IL: Southern Illinois University Press, 1969.

Weiss analyzes sport while comparing and contrasting the perceptions of other authors such as Huizinga, Callois, Dewey, and others on related areas of sport. In some ways this is a history of philosophical development in sport and of those who have contributed to this discussion. He examines thoroughly all components of sport while raising questions and concerns about sport and its relationship to other subjects.

Dissertations

C-18. **Dissertation Abstracts International**. Ann Arbor, MI: University Microfilms. 1938- . Online and CD-ROM formats available.

This comprehensive source lists doctoral dissertations published around the world in many different subject areas, many of which relate to sport and sport science. (See entries A-37, B-19, and D-13.)

C-19. **Health, Physical Education and Recreation Microform Publications Bulletin**. Eugene, OR: University of Oregon, 1949- . 5 issues/yr.

This bulletin from the College of Human Development and Performance is published every five years with two supplements published in between at one year intervals. It provides access to thesis and dissertation listings for works published in physical education, health, recreation, and the related areas of leisure and sport. Many of the listings are available in microfilm format. A select number of out-of-print or difficult to obtain materials are also listed. (See entry B-20.)

Bibliographies and Catalogs

The bibliographies listed here are useful in identifying and locating material in various subject areas related to sport and sports science. Bibliographies often include overviews or brief discussions of research involved in those subject areas.

C-20. Davis, Lenwood, comp. **Black Athletes in the United States: A Bibliography of Books, Articles, Autobiographies, and Biographies on Black Professional Athletes in the United States, 1800-1981**. Westport, CT: Greenwood Press, 1982.

Davis's work cites the involvement of African-American athletes in the sports of baseball, basketball, boxing, football, golf, and tennis in the United States. He includes chapters on major and general reference books, major and general African-American reference books, books by African-American athletes, books about African-American athletes, and listings of article citations. Several helpful appendices are included, one listing halls of fame. Very brief annotations are made for monographs. A total of 3,871 citations are included.

C-21. Lenskyj, Helen, ed. **Women, Sport and Physical Activity: Research and Bibliography**. Ottawa, Canada: Government of Canada, Fitness and Amateur Sport, 1988.

This is a bilingual resource that provides over 1,200 book and journal article citations. Selection was based on specific criteria within gender and sport; one of the editor's objectives was to formulate the bibliography excluding articles that contain gender-related or sexist bias. Each chapter is composed of an essay and a bibliographic listing of sources; a suggested reading list is provided in the conclusion of each chapter with key resources noted. A solid introduction to feminist theory, sport, culture and society, psychological and physiological considerations, exercise and reproductive functions completes the volume. All citations come from the SPORT Database (entry B-43). Emphasis is on North American literature with Canadian authors dominating the source listing. The second edition will be available in 1992.

C-22. Redekop, Paul. **Sociology of Sport: An Annotated Bibliography**. New York: Garland Press, 1988.

This bibliography is composed primarily of English-language citations published from 1960-85 in journal articles, books, and chapters within books. Textbooks and dissertations are not included. Redekop divides this book into seven chapters: theory and method in sociology of sport; sport and culture; sport and society; socialization, sport, and sex roles; minority relations; race/handicapped; deviance and sport; violence, spectators, and fans; and drug use. An author index is provided. Approximately three-quarters of the 579 citations are annotated.

C-23. Shoebridge, Michele. **Women in Sport: A Selected Bibliography**. London: Mansell, 1988.

This very useful resource updates and complements Remley's *Women in Sport* (entries C-7 and C-8). Journal articles listed cover the years 1970-86. Only English-language publications are included. Monographs and conference papers are cited from 1900; their scope is international and some annotations are included. Cited theses are primarily from North America. In general, this bibliography is international in coverage, with the majority of citations coming from the United Kingdom. Compared to Remley, this source expands the variety of subject coverage to include ethnic groups, the disabled, and topics in sport sciences. Each chapter is broken down by subject and then by type of material (monograph, thesis, etc.). There is no title index.

C-24.   **Sport Bibliography**. Champaign, IL: Human Kinetics, 1986- . Annual.
This is a series (to date there are ten numbers) of specialized bibliographies available from the Sport Information Resource Centre (SIRC). The subject-specific categories include the following:

1.   Ethics in Sport

2.   Spectator Violence

3.   Pierre de Coubertin

4.   Commercialization of Amateur Sport

5.   Physical Fitness in the Third Age

6.   Physical Activity and Mental Health

7.   Employee Fitness

8.   Sport Violence

9.   Nutrition and Physical Activity

10.   Aquatic Management

A table of contents focusing on subject divisions relevant to the topic is provided for each category and each bibliography contains more than 200 citations, most of which are annotated. The scope of resources includes books, book chapters, conference proceedings, periodicals, theses, and microforms. Citations follow standard SIRC format. (See entry B-22.)

C-25.   Stark, Richard W., ed. **Sport and Recreation for the Disabled: A Bibliography 1984-1989**. Gloucester, Canada: Sport Information Resource Centre, 1989.
This is a current bibliography dealing with sport and the disabled athlete. It is the third bibliography on the subject produced by the staff at SIRC. Aside from the occasional bibliographies appearing in various journals, this is the best paper resource for locating materials on this subject. More than 4,000 citations derived from the SPORT Database (entry B-43) are included. Very comprehensive subject access from general to specific information is provided. The scope of coverage extends to administration of programs, facilities planning, and leisure activities coordination. Abstracts for all the citations are provided, and the audience level is identified.

C-26.   University of Illinois at Urbana-Champaign. Applied Life Studies Library. **Dictionary Catalog of the Applied Life Studies Library**. 4 vol., 2 suppl. Boston: G. K. Hall, 1977, 1982.
This catalog lists over 19,500 books and microfilms available in the University of Illinois, Urbana-Champaign Applied Life Sciences Library. Special emphasis is on sport sciences and leisure study. Internal dissertations at the master's and doctoral levels are arranged in alphabetical order. The catalog uses Library of Congress subject headings and Dewey Decimal System call numbers.

C-27.   Zucker, Harvey Marc, and Lawrence J. Babich. **Sport Films: A Complete Reference**. Jefferson, NC: McFarland, 1987.

Zucker's work contains 2,042 citations of sports films. The scope of film topics ranges from spectator sports to the integral part that sport plays in certain movies. Title of film, release date, film location, running time, producer, and annotations are all provided. The films are broken down into major sporting categories. Also provided are chapters dealing with athletes in films and actors' portrayals of famous athletes. A selected bibliography, general index, and title index are provided.

Dictionaries

Dictionaries of sport, like other topic-specific works, contain information about the spelling, pronunciation, usage, and sometimes the background of works and/or persons related to the field of sports.

C-28.   Porter, David L., ed. **Biographical Dictionary of American Sports**. 4 vols. New York: Greenwood Press, 1977-87.

This set was compiled into four volumes that can be purchased separately or together. The first two volumes are subject specific to the sports of baseball and football; the last two cover outdoor and indoor sports of all kinds. All volumes concentrate on American athletes only. The format for the entries in each volume includes a biographical note with its own bibliography. At the end of each volume there is a signed author profile. Appendices vary in each volume.

> C-28A.   **Biographical Dictionary of American Sports. Baseball**. New York: Greenwood Press, 1987.
>
> This volume lists 500 baseball entries from post-Revolutionary War time to 1986. The length of the biographical entries ranges from 300 to 900 words, depending on the fame of the individual covered.

> C-28B.   **Biographical Dictionary of American Sports. Football**. New York: Greenwood Press, 1987.
>
> This volume presents 520 biographies of individuals involved with the sport of football from 1870 to 1987. As in the previous volume, the length of the entries ranges from 300 to 900 words, depending on the fame of the individual.

> C-28C.   **Biographical Dictionary of American Sports. Outdoor Sports**. New York: Greenwood Press, 1989.
>
> This volume contains 519 entries that cover a broad spectrum of interests: auto racing, golf, horse racing, lacrosse, skiing, soccer, speedskating, tennis, and track and field. The communications section includes writers, commentators, sportscasters, and promoters. The miscellaneous category includes amateur sport administrators, bicyclists, bobsledders, equestrian riders, field hockey players, rodeo participants, rowers, softball players, as well as participants in water polo and yachting competitions. The appendices provide helpful information on horses, people, events, organizations, and periodicals cited in this volume.

C-28D. **Biographical Dictionary of American Sports. Basketball and Other Indoor Sports**. New York: Greenwood Press, 1989.

Porter includes more than 550 biographical entries. Indoor sports include bowling, diving, gymnastics, ice hockey, swimming, weight lifting, and wrestling. The miscellaneous section lists people, places (including Olympic sites), associations, and periodical citations.

C-29. **Webster's Sport Dictionary**. Springfield, MA: G. C. Merriam Co., 1976.

This dictionary is geared to the average sports fan with a listing of over 8,800 words that are commonly used by players, broadcasters, sportswriters, or found in rule books. In the dictionary, multiple term usages are differentiated by sport. Hunting and fishing terms are included in the broad context of the sporting world.

Encyclopedias

In sport as in most topical information areas there are two basic types of encyclopedias. General encyclopedias incorporate a full range of subject areas and often provide a quick overview of each topic. Specialized encyclopedias are more devoted to specific subject coverage. A word of caution might be added here. In the sport literature, the word "encyclopedia" used in a title can be misleading. Sports encyclopedias often are not true encyclopedias; they often record only individual and overall statistics rather than providing a written overview of the history and development of a particular sport. For example, *The Baseball Encyclopedia* provides excellent coverage of players and league statistics but very little written text.

C-30. American College of Sports Medicine. **Encyclopedia of Sport Sciences and Medicine**. New York: Macmillan, 1971.

The *Encyclopedia of Sport Sciences and Medicine* is the most comprehensive sports medicine book to date. There is even an important section on the history and development of sport medicine. The book is divided into eleven areas:

1. physical activity — general
2. physical activity — sports
3. games and exercises
4. environment
5. emotions and intellect
6. growth, development, and aging
7. drugs
8. prevention and injury
9. special applications of physical activity to the handicapped individual
10. rehabilitation
11. safety and protection

Within each area, from four to seven subchapters follow relevant issues. Each article under these subheadings is signed by a subject specialist. Lists of references are also included in these articles. All sports for both sexes are covered. There is a usable subject and author index.

C-31.　Cureton, Thomas K., Jr. **Encyclopedia of Physical Education. Fitness and Sports**. 4 vols. Reston, VA: American Alliance for Health, Physical Education, Recreation and Dance, 1977- .

In this set each volume follows a similar format. There are different volume editors, section editors, and individual authors — usually all professionals in the fields of physical education, fitness, and/or sports.

C-31A.　Vol. 1. Bosco, James S., ed. **Philosophy, Programs, and History** (1981).

Bosco clearly presents the philosophy, aims, and objectives of sport in this volume. A good introduction to the history and development of sport programs affiliated with schools, the military, and related organizations.

C-31B.　Vol. 2. Stull, G. Alan, ed. **Training, Environment, Nutrition, and Fitness** (1980).

Stull focuses on the environmental aspects of physical performance, the nutritional aspects of training and physical performance, and differences between youth and adult fitness.

C-31C.　Vol. 3. Frost, Ruben, ed. **Sports, Dance and Related Activities** (1977).

In this volume Frost covers the origins of each sport and traces its growth, advances, present status, and affiliations with other sports. The nature of the sport, its fundamental skills, and other important aspects of the sport are discussed as well. Good background is provided covering the differences between men's and women's sports; good examples are given for basketball and lacrosse. Each article is written by a person or persons knowledgeable in the field.

C-31D.　Vol. 4. Cureton, Thomas K., Jr., ed. **Human Performance: Efficiency and Improvements in Sports, Exercise and Fitness** (1985).

Cureton contributes the sport science volume of the set. This work analyses and discusses measurements and other tests involved in sport sciences.

C-32.　Diagram Group. **Rule Book, the Authoritative Up-to-Date Illustrated Guide to the Regulations, History, and Object of All Major Sports**. New York: St. Martin's Press, 1983.

C-33.　Hickok, Ralph. **New Encyclopedia of Sports**. New York: McGraw Hill, 1977.

This has been an important title in most sports collection. It defines sport as a physical activity and does not include the topic of games. Each sport has its own entry. Some historical essays and a variety of entries on specialized areas within specific sports are included. Hickok includes basic techniques with diagrams. An example is automobile racing, where he covers extensively the history of racing, lists various races, differentiates between the varieties of racing, and provides a glossary of terms used in the sport. There is no index.

C-34. Knuttgen, H. G. **Olympic Book of Sports Medicine**. Boston: Blackwell Scientific, 1988.

This resource is an International Olympic Committee publication produced in collaboration with the International Federation of Sport Medicine. It covers the major aspects of sport medicine including chapters on the treatment of injuries, injury prevention, performance assessment, nutrition, performance enhancement, optimal performance, and research measurements. A helpful index completes the volume.

C-35. Menke, Frank Grant. **The Encyclopedia of Sports**. 6th ed. South Brunswick, NJ: A. S. Barnes and Co., 1978.

This volume is related to Ralph Hickok's *New Encyclopedia of Sports* (see entry C-33) but is not as complete.

C-36. White, Jess R., ed. **Sports Rules Encyclopedia**. Champaign, IL: Leisure Press, 1990.

White reproduces rules for over fifty-two sports, mostly those involved in the Olympics. He gives association information regarding the rules for each sport and their application and provides a suggestion list of relevant periodicals. This volume complements the Diagram Group's comprehensive *Rule Book* (see entry C-32).

Directories

C-37. **Blue Book of College Athletics**. Akron, OH: Rohrich Corp., 1989- .

This work represents a combination of two important directories in the sports literature, the *Blue Book of Senior Colleges and Universities* and the *Blue Book of Junior and Community Colleges*. This is the book to use for information about names of athletic programs, campus sporting facilities, athletic coaches of both sexes, sport information directors, and conference and division memberships.

C-38. **NAIA Membership and District Directory**. Kansas City, MO: National Association of Intercollegiate Athletics. Annual.

C-39. **National Directory of College Athletics (Men's Edition)**. Amarillo, TX: R. Franks Publishing Ranch, 1976-77- . Annual.

C-40. **National Directory of College Athletics (Women's Edition)**. Amarillo, TX: R. Franks Publishing Ranch, 1976-77- . Annual.

C-41. **NCAA Directory**. Mission, KS: National Collegiate Athletics Association, 1976- . Annual.

C-42. **NSGA Buying Guide**. Mount Prospect, IL: National Sporting Goods Association, 1974/75- . Annual.

Known as the "yellow pages of the sporting goods industry," this guide provides information on major suppliers, manufacturers' representatives, and associations. A product-reference index and a category of resources section allows for quick access to specific sports equipment. This directory includes the supplier's name, address, phone number, watts/telex number, and the name of the firm's president and/or a national sales manager where applicable.

C-43. Soderberg, Paul, Helen Washington, and Jaques Cattell Press, comps. **The Big Book of Halls of Fame in the United States and Canada: Sports**. New York: R. R. Bowker, 1977- .

Arranged by individual sport, this book lists specific halls of fame and inductees. Various levels of competition—high school, state, and college—are included. A brief history of each hall of fame is presented; address and specific list of names are included. An interesting three-part trivia section (trivia classified, year index, and trivia index) provides sport information classified under five major headings. A separate index to all information is provided.

C-44. **Sports Market Place 1990**. Princeton, NJ: Sportsguide Master Reference, 1984- . Annual.

Sports Market Place replaces *Sportsguide Master Reference* and continues as the most complete resource in providing all kinds of sport information to the researcher. Chapters are divided by specific sport, multisport professional/trade associations, college athletic organizations, multisport publishers, TV/radio broadcasters and programmers, promotion/event athletic management services, market data/directories/information services, trade show/meetings calendar, college/university sport degrees, suppliers, sales agents, and firm names. Indices include multisport, brand trade name, and geographical location. This work is viewed by the profession as "the directory of directories" for sport. The 1990 edition contains over 760 pages and incorporates all aspects of sport from association publications to sporting goods manufacturers. Another useful feature is a listing of academic degrees available in sport management. The promotion/event/athlete management section provides subject access to the scope of services as well as company information, including contact person, address, phone number, and company description.

Indexes, Abstracts, and Databases

Related indexes in the area of sport include but are not limited to *Current Index to Journals in Education* (*CIJE*) (entry A-52), *Psychological Abstracts* (entry A-57), and *Sociological Abstracts* (entry A-60), which have been covered in other chapters of this book. More specific titles focusing on individual sport topics include the following:

C-45. **Completed Research in Health, Physical Education, Recreation and Dance**. Reston, VA: Research Consortium of the American Alliance for Health, Physical Education, Recreation and Dance (AAHPERD), 1959- . Annual.

This work is an index to abstracts, bibliographies, and institution reports. Arranged alphabetically by university and by author's last name, it is a helpful and informative source in the field of sport. Theses are also listed and many have abstracts. The number of issues fluctuates. A bibliography is provided, which contains a listing of published research in related areas, monographs, and serial citations. Citations are listed in alphabetical order.

C-46. **Index Medicus**. Washington, DC: National Library of Medicine, New Series, 1960- . Available through DIALOG, BRS, and in CD-ROM format.

Begun in 1916 under the title *Quarterly Cumulative Index to Current Medical Literature*, this resource provides access to the biomedical journal literature. The coverage is relevant to the sports sciences. "Original journal articles are indexed as well as those letters, editorials, biographies, and obituaries that have substantive contents," say the publication's editors. The terminology is controlled through Medical Subject Headings (MeSH), which are updated and revised yearly. A monthly bibliography entitled "Bibliography of Medical Reviews" is included in every issue.

C-47.   **Leisure, Recreation and Tourism Abstracts**. Farnham Royal, United Kingdom: Commonwealth Agricultural Bureaux, 1975- . Quarterly. Available online.

The *LRTA* makes it possible to examine quickly and easily the contents of journal articles and chapters within books; all abstracts are provided in English. It provides very general subject headings that are coded and allows for more specific terminology — even down to geographical region. Although primarily a British resource, sections on sport and recreation receive worldwide coverage. Many North American journal articles on sport information are also included. (See entries A-55 and D-25.)

C-48.   **Physical Education Index**. Cape Girardeau, MO: Ben Oak, 1978- . Quarterly, with the fourth issue a bound hardcover cumulation.

Physical Education Index provides good subject coverage of almost 200 periodicals in areas related to sport and physical education and of research done in those areas. The majority of citations are in English but English abstracts of foreign publications are included as well. Coverage consists of physical education, dance, physical therapy, sports participation and sport sciences, and other related areas. *Physical Education Index* includes book reviews, articles discussing pertinent legislation, reports of national and international associations, and information about outstanding professionals in the field. This index does not include calendar or job opening information, editorials, letters, election reports, or other short-term miscellany. (See entry B-42.)

C-49.   **Sport and Leisure: A Journal of Social Science Abstracts**. Specialized Information Retrieval and Library Services (SIRLS). Waterloo, Canada: University of Waterloo Press, 1980-91. 3 issues/yr.

Previously titled *Sociology of Leisure and Sport Abstracts*, this source provides access to articles related to sport and leisure in current journals, published conference proceedings, and monographic sources. Resources included are systematically searched for scholarly research articles pertaining to the social sciences and their relationship to the scientific study of sport and leisure activities. The entire range of the social sciences is included. This resource is invaluable as an access point to previously unpublished papers. Government documents, theses, chapters from books, and some foreign language materials are also included. Format includes a complete bibliographical description as well as an abstract for each citation. Author, subject, and source indexes are included. As of 1991 this publication was temporarily suspended.

Core Journals

Because of the wide range of sport interests represented in the periodical literature, the journal entries have been grouped by specific category to better facilitate subject access.

Physical Education

C-50.   **Adapted Physical Activity Quarterly**. Champaign, IL: Human Kinetics, 1984- .
Quarterly. Indexed in *Physical Education Index*, *Psychology Abstracts*, *Sport Documentation*.

Its editors call this publication a "multidisciplinary journal designed to stimulate and communicate scholarly inquires related to physical activities for special populations." It is an excellent resource providing extensive information across a broad spectrum of applied physical education interests. It includes reviews of equipment and facilities and discusses methodologies in physical education; and it presents ideas for creative activities in the field. (See entry B-44.)

C-51.   **Journal of Physical Education, Recreation and Dance**. Reston, VA: American Alliance for Health, Physical Education, Recreation and Dance, 1981- . Monthly. Indexed in *Cumulative Index to Journals in Education*, *Education Index*, and *Physical Education Index*.

The members of the American Alliance for Health, Physical Education, Recreation and Dance (AAHPERD) use this journal to locate and follow recent events in their fields and to define current issues related to physical education, recreation, and dance. Regular departments appear in each number. New procedures are frequently discussed, book reviews are presented, and abstracts accompany articles. There is a Canadian equivalent to this title, Canadian Association for Health, Physical Education and Recreation/l'Association Canadienne pour la Santé, l'Éducation Physique et Loisir. (See entry B-51.)

C-52.   **Journal of Teaching in Physical Education (JTEP)**. Champaign, IL: Human Kinetics, 1981- . Quarterly. Indexed in *Cumulative Index to Journals in Education* and *Physical Education Index*.

Published mainly for students, teachers, teacher/educators, and administrators in physical education, this publication presents all aspects of activities related to physical education plus a wide spectrum of related articles. Research articles, descriptive studies, surveys, review articles, and discussions appear in the course of a publication year. (See entry B-51.)

C-53.   **SportSearch**. Ottawa, Canada: Sport Information Resource Centre, 1985- . Monthly. Available through DIALOG, BRS, CAN/OLE, DIMDI, and Data Star services. CD-ROM format is *SPORT Discus*.

This journal and database is the most internationally comprehensive index dealing with all of sport. In 1988 however, beginning with volume 4, the format was changed to support use as a current awareness index. Over 300 sport-related periodicals (primarily English-language titles) are now included; beginning with the March, 1990, issue, abstracts were added. Relevant articles from nonsport journals are also included. In addition, books, book chapters, congresses, proceedings, and other publications are identified. This publication indirectly supplants *Sport and Recreation Index* and *Sport and Fitness Index* and can function as a paper backup to the *SPORT Discus*. The *SPORT Discus* database also provides a comprehensive index to the Microform Publications Collection of the International Institute for Sport and Human Performance.

Sport Sciences

C-54. **American Journal of Sports Medicine**. Baltimore, MD: Williams and Wilkins/ Orthopaedic Society for Sports Medicine, 1972- . Bimonthly. Indexed in *Current Contents/Clinical Medicine, Cumulative Index to Nursing and Allied Health Literature, Education Index, Index Medicus, Physical Education Index*, and *SportSearch*.

This is a publication with a wide range of topics, whose audience is medical personnel involved with sport. The majority of articles focus on the cause and effect of sport injuries. An average of fifteen articles appear in each issue and an abstract is provided for each. Supplements are published as special issues.

C-55. **Canadian Journal of Sports Sciences**. Downsview, Canada: University of Toronto, 1976- . Quarterly. Formerly *Canadian Journal of Applied Sports Sciences*. Indexed in *Biological Abstracts, Chemical Abstracts, Index Medicus*, and *SportSearch*.

This is the official research publication of the Canadian Association of Sport Sciences. This journal's abstracts are printed in both English and in French. Emphasis is upon the sport sciences such as exercise physiology and biomechanics, with original research data and book reviews often accompanying the articles.

C-56. **Exercise and Sport Sciences Reviews**. American College of Sports Medicine, 1973- . Annual. Indexed in *Index Medicus* and *SportSearch*.

This periodical reviews current research in social sport and sport science. The range of topics covered is broad; example areas include biochemistry, motor control problems, the sociology of sport, rehabilitation, and epidemiology. Articles are lengthy. A list of contributors with addresses is included.

C-57. **International Journal of Sport Biomechanics**. Champaign, IL: Human Kinetics, 1985- . Quarterly. Indexed in *Physical Education Index, Current Contents/ Clinical Medicine*, and *SportSearch*.

The official journal of the International Society of Biomechanics, *International Journal of Biomechanics* is endorsed by the International Olympic Committee's prestigious Medical Commission and focuses on issues affecting human movement. The journal publishes regular reviews of current publications in the sports literature and provides a section in each issue entitled "research digest" in which brief abstracts from a variety of related journals are provided. Special issues are published sporadically; each is devoted to one specific topic within this broad field.

C-58. **Medicine and Science in Sports and Exercise**. Madison, WI: American College of Sports Medicine, 1969- . Monthly. Indexed in *Current Contents/Clinical Medicine, Exerpta Medica, Index Medicus, Physical Education Index, Psychological Abstracts, Science Citation Index*, and *SportSearch*.

The major thrust of this publication is the presentation of articles related to original technical research in sports medicine. Review articles are included. Emphasis is upon new developments in the field, and the publication is geared to exercise physiologists, physical therapists, and professionals working in the areas of sports medicine.

C-59. **Physician and Sportmedicine**. Minneapolis, MN: McGraw Hill, 1973- . Monthly. Indexed in *Current Contents/Clinical Medicine, Exerpta Medica, Index Medicus, Physical Education Index, Psychological Abstracts,* and *Science Citation Index.*

Articles in this publication cover a great variety of topics of interest to practitioners. Prevention and treatment of sport injuries, athletic conditioning, and fitness are examples of the variety of topics. Reviews and special topics are included.

C-60. **Research Quarterly for Exercise and Sport**. Washington, DC: Alliance for Health, Physical Education, Recreation and Dance, 1930- . Quarterly. Formerly *Research Quarterly*. Indexed in *Current Contents/Clinical Medicine, Exerpta Medica, Index Medicus, Physical Education Index, Psychological Abstracts, Science Citation Index,* and *SportSearch.*

This publication is dedicated to presenting articles about the teaching and researching of physical education. Often the editors focus on a special topic and devote the entire number to it. Book reviews are included.

Social Sport

C-61. **Aethlon: Journal of Sport Literature**. San Diego, CA: San Diego Press, 1983- . Semiannual. Formerly *Arete*. Indexed in *SportSearch.*

Aethlon is a scholarly journal published for the Sports Literature Association that focuses on creative literature of the world of sport. It provides examples of fiction and poetry, essays, and — frequently — reviews of current works.

C-62. **Athletic Administration**. Cleveland, OH: Bashian, 1966- . Bimonthly. Indexed in *Physical Education Index* and *SportSearch.*

This publication covers all administrative aspects of sports from the interscholastic level to the professional level. Articles may be theoretical or practical in nature and may appeal to professional athletic administrators.

C-63. **Athletic Business**. Cleveland, OH: Bashian, 1966- . Monthly. Indexed in *Physical Education Index* and *SportSearch.*

Geared to those involved in administering athletics programs and those whose primary responsibility is the supervision of recreational facilities and fitness centers, this publication provides theoretical and practical advice with a business perspective. Special annual issues are produced in February (The Buyers Guide) and in June (Architectural Showcase Issue).

C-64. **Journal of Sport and Social Issues**. Boston: Northeastern Center for the Study of Sport in Society, 1977- . Semiannual. Indexed in *Leisure, Recreation and Tourism Abstracts, Physical Education Index, Sociological Abstracts,* and *SportSearch.*

Subtitled "The Official Journal of the Center for the Study of Sport in Society, Northeastern University," this publication primarily contains papers presented at various conferences. Abstracts and author affiliations are provided.

C-65. **Journal of Sport History**. Radford, VA: North American Society for Sport History, 1974- . Quarterly. Indexed in *Historical Abstracts* and *SportSearch*.

A scholarly journal published primarily for sport historians. It contains articles, essays, book reviews, and surveys related to the field of sports.

C-66. **Journal of Sport Management**. Champaign, IL: Human Kinetics, 1987- . Semiannual. Indexed in *Physical Education Index*.

This publication is the official journal of the North American Society for Sport Management. Theoretical and practical aspects of management in sport, exercise, dance, and play are its main focus. Research and scholarly articles, book reviews, and abstracts are included. The editors encourage submission of articles covering all perspectives of sport management in all settings.

C-67. **Journal of the Philosophy of Sport**. Champaign, IL: Human Kinetics, 1974- . Annual. Indexed in *Current Contents/Social/Behavioral Sciences*, *Physical Education Index*, *Philosopher's Index*, *Social Science Citation Index*, and *SportSearch*.

Published by the Philosophic Society for the Study of Sport, this journal provides international coverage of the treatment of sport, games, play, dance, and other related human movement endeavors. It is a forum for scholars to exchange insights on the theory of sports. No abstracts for articles are provided.

C-68. **Sociology of Sport Journal**. Champaign, IL: Human Kinetics, 1984- . Quarterly. Indexed in *Physical Education Index*, *Sociological Abstracts*, and *SportSearch*.

Sociology of Sport Journal contains book reviews, important articles, research notes and comments, review essays, and annotated bibliographies from the SIRLS database.

C-69. **The Sport Psychologist**. Champaign, IL: Human Kinetics, 1987- . Quarterly. Indexed in *Physical Education Index*, *Psychological Abstracts*, and *Sociological Abstracts*.

This is the official journal of the International Society of Sport Psychology. It is produced for the use of educational and clinical sport psychologists and others who are interested in various psychological techniques relevant to sports. International in scope, it prints articles related to applied research and professional practice. Profiles of important individuals in the field, a bulletin board, and book and video reviews are provided in each issue.

Miscellaneous

C-70. **Olympic Review: Official Publication of the Olympic Movement**. Lausanne, Switzerland: International Olympic Committee, 1894- . Bimonthly. Indexed in *Physical Education Index* and *Sport and Leisure: A Journal of Social Science Abstracts*.

News items relating to the national/international federations, the governing bodies, and the committees of the Olympic movement are presented in this official publication. It features the latest happenings in the world of Olympic sport and in any areas that relate to activities of the movement.

C-71. **Referee: The Magazine of Sports Officials**. Franksville, WI: Mano Enterprises, 1976- . Monthly. Indexed in *Physical Education Index*.

This title is designed specifically for professional referees and others involved with sports officiating. Topics often highlighted include the legal and psychological aspects of sports. Specific sections cover baseball, softball, soccer, football, basketball, and volleyball.

C-72. **Women's Sports and Fitness**. Palo Alto, CA: Women's Sport Publishing, 1979- . Indexed in *SportSearch*.

Although this popular magazine focuses on the image of women in sports, other related topics are presented in depth. One of its most interesting sections is "My Sport," a feature that profiles women who participate regularly in a specific sport.

Conference Proceedings

There are a wide variety of national and international sport organizations that produce conference publications; many appear irregularly. Many of these publications are indexed in the SPORT Database (see entry B-43). Other publications remain illusive. It is often necessary to contact organizations directly to verify conference information. Several important regular information providers include the following:

C-73. **Conference Proceedings and Reports, Games of the Olympiad**. New York: United States Olympic Association.

Irregularly published by the Association, this publication presents documentation of various meetings and activities of various committees.

C-74. **Proceedings and Newsletter. North American Society for Sport History**. University Park, PA: North American Society for Sport History, 1973- .

Focusing on physical education and training as well as sport history, these proceedings provide coverage of the Society's presentations, activities, and meetings.

C-75. **Proceedings of the Convention. National Collegiate Athletic Association**. 60th- . Los Angeles, CA: 1965/66- .

Another important source providing information on athletic clubs and collegiate sports in the United States.

C-76. **Proceedings of the Special Convention. National Collegiate Athletic Association**. Chicago: 1973- .

Also called *NCAA Special Convention Proceedings*, this publication provides information on the activities of special NCAA congresses, the first of which was held in August, 1973.

Statistical Sources

C-77.   **American Statistics Index**. Bethesda, MD: Congressional Information Service, 1973- . Monthly, with annual cumulations. Online and CD-ROM formats available.

This source provides access to information produced in over 500 federal government agencies. Information relating to sport and sport activities is included. Access is through a comprehensive index published separately from the abstracts. Subjects, names, and categories act as points of access to this large pool of American statistical data. (See entries A-79 and D-53.)

C-78.   Carruth, Gorton, and Eugene Ehrlich. **Facts and Dates of American Sports: From Colonial Days to the Present**. New York: Harper & Row, 1988.

This book is a combination chronology, almanac, and recorded fact resource. It follows major sporting events from their inception. The time period covered is 1540 to 1988. Abbreviated bibliographies are provided for famous players, and major memorable sporting events are highlighted in concise paragraphs. The volume also provides several helpful lists of events and winning teams. The indexing is by athlete name, event name, and date.

C-79.   **The ... Information Please Sports Almanac**. Boston: Houghton Mifflin, 1989- . Annual.

For fast reference to all types of sport and sport-related questions requiring statistical information, this is an excellent resource. A year in review (month by month) calendar is followed by a preview calendar of future events. Major sports of baseball, basketball, and football—both collegiate and professional—have individual chapters. Other sports are covered in less detail. This monograph incorporates overviews and statistical information into a quick ready-reference resource for all types of users.

C-80.   Whittingham, Richard. **Rand McNally Sports Places Rated, Ranking American Best Places to Enjoy Sports**. Chicago: Rand McNally, 1986.

Similar in nature to Rand McNally's *Places Rated Almanac*, this unique resource critiques 113 places to visit by applying various criteria, including the presence of major sporting facilities. Each chapter has five sections, each with an introduction providing background. The use of scoring methodology is discussed, a profile of score and rank is given, an alphabetical listing of rank is provided, and a "Top Ten" list is given. The chapters start with pro sports (football, baseball, basketball, hockey, and soccer) and then list college sports (football, men's and women's basketball). These are followed by sports events/facilities, including information about events held, stadiums, arenas, tracks, halls of fame, and frontons.

NOTES

[1]H. Graves, "A Philosophy of Sport," *Contemporary Review*, 78 (December 1900): 878.

[2]John W. Loy, "The Nature of Sport: A Definitional Effort," *Quest*, 10 (May 1968): 1.

[3]John W. Loy, Barry D. McPherson, and Gerald Kenyon, *Sport and Social Systems* (Reading, MA: Addison-Wesley, 1978), 21.

[4]Loy, "The Nature of Sport," 6.

[5]Paul Weiss, *Sport: A Philosophic Inquiry* (Carbondale, IL: Southern Illinois University Press, 1969), 33.

[6]Harold J. VanderZwaag, *Toward a Philosophy of Sport* (Reading, MA: Addison-Wesley, 1972), 34.

[7]Stephen K. Figler, *Sport and Play in American Life: A Textbook in the Sociology of Sport* (Philadelphia, PA: Saunders College, 1981), 8.

[9]Ibid., 9.

[10]Ibid., 10.

[11]Ibid., 12.

[12]D. Stanley Eitzen and George H. Sage, *Sociology of American Sport* (Dubuque, IA: William C. Brown, 1978), 117.

[13]Ronald A. Smith, *Sport and Freedom: The Rise of Big Time College Athletics* (New York: Oxford University Press, 1988), 4.

[14]John Krout, *Annals of American Sport*, vol. 15 of *Pageant of America* (New Haven, CT: Yale University Press, 1929), 185.

[15]Figler, 85.

[16]Eitzen and Sage, 118.

[17]Figler, 118.

[18]Jack W. Berryman, "The Rise of Highly Organized Sports for Preadolescent Boys, 2-15," in *Children in Sport*, Richard A. Magill, Michael J. Ash, and Frank L. Smoll (Champaign, IL: Human Kinetics, 1982).

[19]Donald Chu, *Dimensions of Sport Studies* (New York: Wiley, 1982), 136.

[20]Foster Rhea Dulles, *America Learns to Play: A History of Recreation* (New York: Appleton-Century-Crofts, 1965), 335.

[21]Benjamin G. Rader, *In Its Own Image: How Television Bias Transformed Sports* (New York: Free Press, 1989), 33.

[22]Benjamin G. Rader, *American Sport from the Age of Folk Games to the Age of Televised Sports*, 2d ed. (Englewood Cliffs, NJ: Prentice-Hall, 1990), 243.

[23]Glenn M. Wong, *Essentials of Amateur Sports Law* (Dover, MA: Auburn House, 1988), 480.

[24]Nand Hart-Nibbring and Clement Cottinghan, *The Political Economy of College Sports* (Lexington, MA: D. C. Heath, 1986), 4.

[25]Ibid., 3.

[26]Arthur J. Johnson and James H. Frey, *Government and Sport: The Public Policy Issues* (Totowa, NJ: Rowan and Allanheld, 1985), 4.

[27]Ibid., 13.

[28]Ibid., 2.

[29]Ibid., 1.

[30]Figler, 244.

[31]Anne Ingram, "SPRINT: A Functional Organization That Served as Advocates for Social Change in Girls and Women's Sports, 1970-82," in *ICHPER/CAPPER World Conference: Towards the 21st Century* (Vancouver, Canada, June 9-13, 1987), 226-29.

[32]Herb Appenzeller and Thomas Appenzeller, *Sports and the Courts* (Charlottesville, VA: Michie, 1980), 58.

[33]Figler, 289.

[34]Wong, 103.

[35]Ibid., 103.

[36]Ibid., 262.

[37]Claudine Sherrill, *Adaptive Physical Education and Recreation: A Multidisciplinary Approach*, 3d ed. (Dubuque, IA: William C. Brown, 1986), 76.

[38]Appenzeller and Appenzeller, 219.

[39]John C. Weistart and Cypn H. Lowell, *The Law of Sports* (Indianapolis, IN: Bobbs-Merrill, 1979).

[40]Johnson and Frey, 13.

[41]Susan L. Greendorfer, "Sport," in *Recreation and Leisure: An Introductory Handbook*, eds. Alan Graefe and Stan Parker (State College, PA: Venture Publishing, 1987).

[42]William H. Freeman, *Physical Education and Sport in a Changing Society*, 3d ed. (New York: Macmillan, 1982), 6-7.

[43]Ibid., 10.

[44]Loy, 257.

4

THE LITERATURE OF TRAVEL/TOURISM

Diane Zabel

INTRODUCTION

What are travel and tourism? Are the words *travel* and *tourism* interchangeable or do they have different connotations? An impromptu survey among friends would probably reveal that the two words mean various things to various people. "Travel" can conjure up images of exotic or romantic destinations like Tahiti and Paris or images of matter of course events such as traveling to a funeral or to the annual family reunion. Travel can be for pleasure or for business or a combination of both. It can be an afternoon excursion to the next town or an extended trip around the world. Travelers can be newlyweds on their honeymoon or a bus load of visiting delegates from another country. The only common thread is that travel is an activity conducted over time and space. "Tourism" also has many meanings. It has sometimes been applied only to traveling for pleasure. The word has frequently implied contempt and derision; no one wants to be labeled a "tourist." Additionally, "tourism" has been used to describe the study of travel and tourists.

There is no agreement among researchers, governmental agencies, or leading travel and tourism organizations about what constitutes tourism or who is a tourist. The word "tourist" emerged in late nineteenth-century Britain to describe young men who completed their education with a Grand Tour of the Continent. But travel, generally defined as making a journey, is an activity that can be traced back to the ancient world. In fact, historians sometimes refer to Herodotus the Greek, a fifth century B.C. traveler who visited Karnak and Persia out of curiosity, as the first tourist.[1] Although the Greeks journeyed to the Olympic Games (first held in 776 B.C.), large scale tourism did not evolve until ancient Imperial Rome.[2] The Pax Romana (27 B.C.-180 A.D.), the two century peace, combined with an extensive road system, aided the development of tourism. Romans traveled to historic sites (including the Seven Wonders of the ancient world), sporting events, festivals, plays, spas, and resorts. However, travel as a leisure activity almost disappeared in the period following the collapse of the Roman Empire. Medieval travel centered around the Crusades and religious pilgrimages. Travel for the sake of education took hold in seventeenth-century Europe. Europeans and Americans popularized travel for health in the eighteenth and nineteenth centuries as they journeyed to spas and health resorts in order to "take the waters." Mass tourism, however, did not occur until the late eighteenth and early nineteenth centuries when the industrial revolution improved transportation with the development of steamboats and railroads and increased prosperity and leisure time. Modern tourism developed as a result of advances in transportation systems (automobiles and airplanes) and the rise of a middle class with discretionary time and income.

The modern day traveler travels at comparative speed and in comfort when compared to travelers of another era, but the reasons why people travel have remained unchanged. Although only one of the ancient wonders survives (the Great Pyramids of Giza), the twentieth-century tourist can visit such natural wonders as the Grand Canyon or such attractions as Graceland, Elvis Presley's home in Memphis. A contemporary anthropologist even equates a trip to Walt Disney World with a pilgrimage.[3] People continue to travel in order to visit friends and relatives, to see places of historic significance, to watch or participate in sports and other entertainments, to attend conventions and meetings, to conduct business, and sometimes simply to get away from it all.

The purpose of travel has sometimes been used as a criterion for defining tourists and tourism. The recognition of tourism as a significant economic activity prompted several organizations to develop definitions. Even in the 1930s, agencies realized that a standard definition was essential in order to make data collection and analysis comparable. The first attempt to provide a technical definition of a tourist was undertaken in 1937 by the League of Nations' Committee of Statistical Experts. This committee adopted the following definition of an international tourist:

> Any person visiting a country, other than that in which he usually resides for a period of at least 24 hours (such as):
>
> - persons travelling for pleasure, for family reasons or for health;
> - persons travelling to meetings, or in a representative capacity of any kind (scientific, administrative, diplomatic, religious, or athletic);
> - persons travelling for business reasons;
> - persons arriving in the course of a sea cruise, even when they stay less than 24 hours.
>
> The Committee specifically excluded from the definition:
>
> - persons arriving, with or without a contract of work, to take up an occupation or engage in any business activity in the country;

- other persons coming to establish a residence in the country;

- students and young persons in boarding establishments or schools;

- residents in a frontier zone and persons domiciled in one country and working in an adjoining country;

- travellers passing through a country without stopping, even if the journey takes more than 24 hours.[4]

This definition is important because it became the basis for subsequent definitions. In 1963 the United Nations held a conference in Rome on international travel and tourism. The definitions formulated at this conference differentiated two categories of travelers: tourists and excursionists. A tourist was described as "any person visiting a country other than in which he has his usual place of residence, for any reason other than following an occupation remunerated from within the country visited."[5] The following characteristics distinguished tourists from excursionists:

1. Tourists: temporary visitors staying at least 24 hours in the country visited and the purpose of whose journey can be classified as (a) leisure, i.e., recreation, holiday, health, study, religion or sport; or (b) business; (c) family; (d) mission; or (e) meeting.

2. Excursionists: temporary visitors staying less than 24 hours in the country visited (including travellers on cruises).[6]

Several international organizations urged countries to adopt the Rome Conference definitions, and many nations and organizations have accepted or modified them. The World Tourism Organization, an international organization that promotes tourism, refined definitions of residents and nonresidents and uses residence of the traveler, length of stay, and purpose of travel as measures for characterizing visitors, tourists, and excursionists.

Distance traveled has sometimes been used as an element in defining travelers. The U.S. Travel Data Center, a national nonprofit research center, measures travel in the United States that involves traveling to places one hundred miles or more away from home. The Center is the chief research arm of the American travel industry and the major source of tourism data in this country. Consequently, its definitions of travel and tourism need to be understood by anyone researching travel and tourism in the United States. The Center approved the following definitions in 1985, which are accepted by the Travel Industry Association of America, a national trade association whose membership includes numerous components of the travel and tourism industry:

1. "Travel Industry"—an interrelated amalgamation of those businesses and agencies which totally or in part provide the means of transport, goods, services, accommodations, and other facilities for travel out of the home-community for any purpose not related to local day-to-day activity.

2. "Travel"—the actions and activities of international and domestic travelers (as defined below) taking trips to places outside their home communities for any purpose except commuting to and from work or attending school.

3. "Tourism"—synonymous with "travel."

4. "International Traveler"—any person visiting a country other than that in which he(she) has his(her) usual place of residence for at least 24 hours but not more than one year, and whose main purpose of visit is other than following an occupation remunerated from within the country visited, and the purpose of whose trip can be classified under one or more of the following categories:

pleasure	business
recreation	commerce
holiday	meeting
sport	conference
religion	convention
shopping	trade show
vacation	health
visiting friends or relatives	study

5. "International Excursionist"—travelers, as defined in 4 above, staying less than 24 hours in the country visited (including cruise passengers).

6. "International Tourist"—synonymous with "international traveler."

7. "Domestic Traveler"—any resident of the United States regardless of nationality who travels to a place 100 miles or more away from home within the U.S. or who stays away from home one or more nights in paid accommodations, and who returns home within twelve months, except commuting to and from work or attending school. This includes trips that can be classified under one or more of the following purpose categories:

pleasure	business
recreation	commerce
holiday	meeting
sport	conference
religion	convention
shopping	trade show
vacation	health
visiting friends or relatives	study

8. "Domestic Excursionist" — any person who travels more than 25 miles away from home one way but less than 100 miles and returns home the same day for any purpose except commuting to and from work or attending school, including trips that can be classified under the categories defined in 7 above.[7]

The terminology used by the U.S. Travel Data Center excludes local travel, the everyday commute to work, and travel for the purpose of school or military service. Notice that its definition of a domestic traveler requires a distance of 100 or more miles or paid accommodations for one or more nights. This criterion of accommodation is in part a reflection of the Center's membership: the American Hotel and Motel Association, the Recreation Vehicle Industry Association, and individual hotel and motel chains are among the Center's corporate members. Moreover, the inclusion of accommodation recognizes that travel frequently involves a stay.

There is a significant body of literature on the definitions of travel and tourism.[8] The lack of uniform terminology exists at the international, national, and regional levels, and there is a lack of consensus among agencies, organizations, and individuals involved in researching travel and tourism. One researcher outlined the problems in Great Britain resulting from an absence of standard definitions.[9] One obvious outcome is that uniform data are not collected.

This writer will regard travel and tourism as synonyms and will consider travel/tourism to be an industry composed of an amalgamation of fragmented services that support a traveler's need for transportation, food, lodging, amusement, and recreation. In an effort to collect consistent data on like industries, the United States federal government devised the Standard Industrial Classification (SIC) scheme. Businesses are assigned a four-digit code representing their principal economic activity. For example, 5812 is the code assigned to restaurants because they constitute eating and drinking places, a type of business listed in the *Standard Industrial Classification Manual*. However, travel/tourism is not represented by a single SIC code. The travel/tourism industry encompasses a wide range of diverse industries: travel agencies, tour operators, airlines, cruise lines, rental cars, bus companies, taxicabs, railroads, hotels, motels, bars, gasoline stations, amusement parks, and attractions. Even this is not an exhaustive list of travel/tourism-related businesses because a tourist may buy film, souvenirs, and make other purchases ranging from suntan oil to groceries. The complexity of researching tourism as an economic activity is difficult at best.

IMPORTANCE AS AN INDUSTRY

Travel/tourism is the third-largest retail industry in the United States. An analysis of 1988 retail sales after taxes by the U.S. Travel Data Center indicates that travel/tourism produced more than $300 billion in sales, being surpassed only by automotive dealers and food stores.[10] The travel/tourism industry is also a major source of employment. Statistical data show that it is the second largest private employer in the United States (only the health service industry is greater) and it generates new jobs faster than other sectors of the economy.[11] It is also dominated by small businesses. In 1982 approximately 98 percent of the firms making up the major components of the industry (transportation, lodging, foodservice, entertainment, recreation) fit the U.S. Small Business Administration's definition of a small business.[12] Surprisingly, the United States government trails behind other nations in spending money to promote tourism, especially in the area of attracting international visitors. In 1985 the United States ranked twenty-fourth in the world in the category of expenditures for tourism development.[13]

Travel/tourism is an important growth industry worldwide, especially in developing countries. In 1985 tourism receipts equaled or exceeded $1 billion in thirty-one countries, with the low per capita income nations of Mexico, China, India, Thailand, Portugal, Brazil, and South Korea among the "tourism billionaires."[14] Tourism is the major industry for several countries of the world. Even the poorest of the poor nations have committed scarce resources to tourism development in an effort to obtain desperately needed foreign currency. Third World countries were the destination of approximately 17 percent of all international tourists in 1982.[15]

IMPACT OF TRAVEL/TOURISM

Travel/tourism has important impacts. The economic, environmental, social, and cultural consequences are both positive and negative. There is a significant volume of literature written by social scientists on the effect of tourism on the host country as well as on the visiting guest.[16] This has even been explored in the popular media. The 1985 film *Witness* depicted (and unintentionally intensified) tourists' perceptions of the Amish in Lancaster County, Pennsylvania, as curiosities. Although tourism can bring economic prosperity, it can also bring overdevelopment and contribute to the loss of an area's uniqueness as strip development occurs. Revenue does not always remain in the local community, especially if hotels, motels, and campgrounds are chain rather than independent operations. Because tourism is frequently a seasonal activity for many regions, communities have to adapt to fluctuations in tourism receipts and cash flow problems. Also, revenue may be unpredictable because tourism is affected by external factors such as the weather, natural disasters, political instability, and acts of terrorism. Even though tourism generates jobs, some critics have argued that many of these are low-paying and short-term due to their seasonal nature. Tourism development also requires major capital investments on the part of host countries. Visitors not only need lodging, food, and entertainment but also must make use of municipal services such as sewage treatment, garbage collection, police and fire protection. While tourists make additional demands on these basic services, they can also negatively impact a community by increasing the cost of living or contributing to escalating real estate prices.

The flow of tourists into a region alters the environment. While it can encourage the preservation of natural and built environments (Yellowstone and Colonial Williamsburg are two examples), it can also result in traffic congestion, pollution, a precarious shift in the ecosystem, and a serious depletion of natural resources. The latter two issues in particular have created controversies over the costs and benefits of developing tourism in Third World countries. Big game is both hunted and artificially protected in Africa. Tourism even contributes to the endangerment of the Amazon rain forest. The implications are startling in the poorest of the poor countries. A study of the problems associated with tourism development in the world's least-developed nations outlines the negative environmental consequences:

> The problem of water supply becomes another limitation.... In the dry season the shortages are such that locals may be rationed to a bucket a day while witnessing tourists casually showering on coming off the beach. A western visitor used to an average utilization of 36 gallons per day (including washing and toilet flushing) places excessive pressure on beleaguered resorts during the dry months of the year.[17]

The preceding example illustrates the incongruous living standards that may distinguish hosts from guests.

Some philosophical benefits of tourism are that it fosters an understanding and appreciation of other cultures. Tourism has even been viewed as a mechanism for achieving world peace. In 1988 representatives from sixty-four nations convened in British Columbia, Canada, to hear sessions on the theme of "Tourism—A Vital Force for Peace."[18] Participants concluded that "tourism has the potential to be the largest peace-time movement in the history of mankind because tourism involves people, their culture, their economies, their traditions, their heritage and their religion."[19] The conference also addressed the conflicts that can arise between hosts and guests. The following are some of the noteworthy recommendations proposed at the conference:

- Future and potential tourists must be pre-acquainted with the destinations they are visiting.

- There should be innovative hospitality and awareness programs in host countries.

- Tourism will not be perceived as contributing to peace unless the problem of achieving an equitable distribution of the economic benefits and costs of tourism to the host country is solved. The host country's standard of living and quality of life must be improved. Therefore, government must take a more active, aggressive and proactive role in ensuring an equitable distribution of benefits and costs, a better balance between supply and demand, and an increase in the local share and retention of benefits.

- A new generation of thinking is required which recognizes that environmental protection and enhancement are essential for a healthy tourism industry.

- There is a need for the adoption of policies of sustainable development; a need for a global system of environmental protection, evaluation and monitoring; a need for community involvement in ecological planning and tourism planning at the local level; and a need to respect local environments—the scale, values, cultures, people being visited, homes and sacred places.

- In order for tourism to reach its potential as a vital force for world peace, we recommend the development of curricula which will increase geographic, cultural and linguistic literacy of students; include the teaching of responsible tourism development and the balance between demand-side and supply-side tourism orientations; and incorporate skills that would avoid friction that would arise between host and guest population.[20]

The exposure to another culture is sometimes contrived. Tourists may get a sanitized version of a culture. Westerners, especially Americans, often demand the amenities of home, giving reality to the stereotype of the "ugly American." This artificial interaction was documented by Barbara Weightman in a fascinating study of package tours to India. The following observations were made about the mass tourist in India:

- In India, the tourist spends a large portion of the tour encapsulated in planes, buses, and cars. This is incongruent with a reality where most people walk, use animal transport or other forms of open vehicles, or trains. Although plane travel allows viewing of patterns not readily apparent from the ground, without guidance, the average mass tourist will not be able to interpret them. While buses and cars allow coverage of more space and exposure to more sights in limited time, the traveler is sensually isolated within the vehicle. Tinted windows cloud otherwise brilliant visual perceptions; air-conditioning eliminates pungent odors; and metallic enclosure combined with engine noise drowns both the melody and cacophony of the Indian soundscape.

- Much time is also spent confined within a hotel, primarily of the deluxe variety. What must it mean to the average Indian when many of the tallest buildings in this land are not offices or financial centers, but rather tourist hotels?

- Enclosure and height exacerbate not only real but also cultural distance already apparent between tourist and host. External spaces, immediate to the hotel, are kept free of beggars and other unfortunates in an effort not only to protect the visitor but also to maintain a good image.

- Restaurants, shops, and entertainment facilities within the hotel encourage the tourist to stay in this pseudo-Indian home away from home. Thus social contact with ordinary people is discouraged.

- Tour destinations tend to have large populations. The most commonly visited are cities of 900,000 to 9,000,000 people. While tourists experience urban settings, about 77 percent of all Indians experience rural ones.... Visits to rural villages ... are virtually nonexistent.

- The package tour insulates, regulates, and prescribes. Cosmopolitanized, homogenized tourist landscapes, designed to provide all the comforts of home, not only clash with the host landscape but also are protective and restrictive. On the tour itself, observation of objects and events are equated with experience. More importantly perhaps, people are portrayed as objects of curiosity on the land, not as integral elements of landscape.[21]

STUDY OF TRAVEL/TOURISM AND ACADEMIC PROGRAMS

Social scientists—particularly geographers, anthropologists, sociologists, and economists—have studied the impacts of tourism. However, the development of travel/tourism as a distinct field of study did not occur until the 1960s and 1970s. The emergence of specialized research journals during this period corresponded to the growth of travel/tourism as a specialized discipline.

Travel/tourism is in its infancy as an academic discipline and is distributed over several programs in colleges and universities. Although travel/tourism exists as a separate academic unit at some institutions, tourism education is more often part of the curricula of leisure studies, recreation and parks, business, hospitality, urban and regional planning, landscape architecture, and geography. Tourism educators are divided over whether tourism studies constitute a distinct or a multidisciplinary academic offering. A 1981 article written by Neil Leiper, an Australian educator, maintained that a multidisciplinary approach to tourism education is fragmented and argued that tourism, although interdisciplinary, is a new and distinct discipline. The author recommended that this scientific discipline be named "tourology"[22] because tourism is an imprecise term. A variation on this theme surfaced in an article published in the late 1980s in an American journal. The authors worried that "the hosting academic unit dictates the nature and direction of the program."[23] The following examples were used to support this contention:

> Programs in recreation and leisure most often focus on attractions and theme parks, outdoor/environmental resource management and, to a lesser extent, economic development. Similarly, hotel and restaurant management programs offering strong resort and casino training and geography programs often send graduates into the travel agency and group tour employment sectors.[24]

Tourism curricula have often been attached to other academic programs because of budget constraints. However, some educators believe that tourism rightly belongs in a social science curriculum because of its interdisciplinary nature, use of empirical research methods, and importance as an area of scholarly research. This acceptance of tourism as an academic study has been gradual. Some academicians, including social scientists, have dismissed tourism as a "frivolous and lightweight"[25] pursuit and have "tended to avoid it in order to maintain their image as serious scholars."[26] In fact, it has been claimed that "tourism was discovered by social scientists in the early 1970s, and has become a legitimate area for systematic investigation."[27] A comparative analysis of articles published in the *Annals of Tourism Research* and the *Journal of Leisure Research* confirms this. Of the 229 articles published in the *Annals of Tourism Research* from 1974 to 1986, 53 articles were written by geographers, 45 by anthropologists, and 33 by economists.[28]

Tourism has relationships to other social sciences: geography, business (especially marketing and advertising), economics, anthropology, sociology, psychology, political science, history, recreation, urban and regional planning, and law. The *Annals of Tourism Research*, a leading scholarly journal, has published special issues focusing on tourism's relationship to sociology, geography, anthropology, political science, social psychology, environmental studies, and leisure and recreation.

Geographers were probably the first social scientists to study tourism. Their interest dates back to the 1930s. Douglas G. Pearce has traced the history of geographical interest in tourism and has noted two early studies conducted by geographers on the economic aspects of tourism. A 1933 article looked at the growth of tourism in mining towns in the Canadian Rockies and a 1945 article examined the role of highway US16 in the development of tourism in South Dakota.[29] Both were published in *Economic Geography*. Physical and cultural geographers have also been interested in tourism because of its environmental and social impacts.

Tourism's linkage to business and economics is obvious because tourism is an economic activity. The field of business views tourism as an industry and is particularly interested in the revenues and jobs that it generates. Market researchers investigate the demographics of travel: who travels where, how, when, and why. Advertisers want to know the best way to reach targeted audiences in order to promote tourism. While business research often focuses on particular segments of the industry, accommodations or transportation for example, economists may study the costs and benefits associated with tourism, tourism's role in Third World economies, or the multiplier effect of tourism revenues (how tourism stimulates a local economy).

The primary interest of anthropologists has been the relationship between hosts and guests. Anthropologists traditionally have regarded tourism as an intrusion upon host societies. An analysis of a 1976 report issued by UNESCO reveals that "while economists were generally positively oriented to tourism as a relatively painless, quick, and labor-intensive avenue to rapid development, sociologists and anthropologists, concerned, or perhaps overconcerned, with the preservation of native cultures and societies, have in the past generally taken a negative attitude towards the industry."[30] This attitude has changed in the past fifteen years as some field work has demonstrated that tourism can also have a beneficial impact on the host society. A 1980 article in the *Annals of Tourism Research* written by Valene L. Smith, an authority on the anthropology of tourism, urged anthropologists and other social scientists to work jointly with industry "in order to analyze both sides of the coin."[31] Smith argued that anthropological studies of national characters (societies' perceptions of other cultures) could be particularly useful in creating a "better understanding between the toured and the touring."[32]

Sociologists have also become increasingly interested in tourism. Like anthropologists, sociologists are interested in the social and cultural consequences of tourism. Sociologists have also recently argued that their unique perspective can offer different interpretations of the host/guest relationship. While anthropologists have generally studied nonwestern and nonindustrialized societies sociologists have concentrated on modern western societies. Sociologists' observations about societal change are also valuable. Demographic trend analysis is an indispensable tool in tourism marketing and planning. Changing demographics impact the demand for tourism-related services. For example, as the baby boomers age, they will contribute to the growth of the tourism industry in the 1990s and beyond, especially because the elderly account for the largest proportion of pleasure travel dollars. The tourism industry will benefit enormously from the rapid growth of retirees in the future.

Social psychology in combination with sociology, marketing, and advertising has been applied to the study of tourism to explain what motivates people to travel. This behavioral science is referred to as psychographics. While demographics classify people by variables such as age, sex, occupation, and income, psychographics classify people by personality traits. Stanley C. Plog, a key proponent of this approach to tourism research, has created two categories of travelers: psychocentrics and allocentrics.[33] Psychocentrics are more comfortable with the familiar while allocentrics enjoy adventurous travel experiences. Psychocentrics drive rather than fly, select touristy destinations, enjoy tourist attractions, opt for fast food rather than more interesting dining experiences, are low energy, and prefer completely arranged package tours. Allocentrics are outgoing, energetic, confident, and look for the exact opposite in a travel experience. The following contrast is a good description of the two types: "Allos tend to accept challenges, meet the residents, try out the food and drink, look for the new experience. The allo would go to China or Nepal; the psychocentric would prefer a nearby state park."[34]

The United States' boycott of the 1980 Summer Olympics is a prime example of the political aspects of tourism. Because governments can place restrictions on travel, tourism can be used as a political weapon. However, governments more commonly play the role of tourism promoters. Successful tourism development generally involves a cooperative effort by government and private industry. It requires a practical knowledge of law, planning, and design, ranging from an understanding of local zoning ordinances to the visa requirements of individual countries. Curiously, political scientists have been the group of social scientists least interested in tourism research. The 1980 Midwest Political Science Meeting was the first American political science conference to include a session on the politics of tourism and a participant recalled that "only two of the participants were political scientists, and the panel members outnumbered the entire audience."[35] In 1983 the *Annals of Tourism Research* published a special thematic issue on tourism and political science. Harry G. Matthews, a political scientist whose research includes tourism in the Caribbean, guest edited the issue and developed the following explanations for the lack of interest on the part of political scientists:

> First, tourism politics seldom contain the seeds of controversy necessary to attract the attention of large numbers of political scientists. In the United States, tourism politics goes scarcely unnoticed by the media and is seldom discussed by politicians. Unlike the politics of abortion, equal rights, the environment, energy, or education — to name only a few examples — tourism politics evokes few strong feelings among established groups of citizens.
>
> Perhaps a second reason that political scientists have paid little attention to tourism is the lack of peer and financial support.... At a typical American university, a political scientist with a scholarly interest in tourism might be looked upon as dabbling in frivolity — not as a serious scholar but as an opportunist looking for a tax-deductible holiday.
>
> Like other social scientists, political scientists probably attain a scholastic interest in tourism through a back door.... Their attention to tourism is likely to be an outgrowth of some other priority. Whatever the case might be, it does appear that interest among political scientists in tourism has been growing, although at a much slower pace than among some other groups of social scientists.[36]

Tourism also has linkages to leisure, recreation, and sport. Travel for pleasure assumes discretionary time, and getting away from it all is a form of recreation. In fact, tourism has to compete with other recreational activities. For example, some people prefer armchair traveling to actually leaving their home. Pleasure travel frequently involves recreational activities ranging from skiing to visiting theme parks. Recreational facilities in turn are an integral part of accommodations. Although tourism's ties to leisure and recreation seem obvious, this relationship has received scant attention by scholars. The *Annals of Tourism Research* explored this connection in a special issue in 1987. A theme throughout the issue was "that leisure and recreation research has proceeded on the one camp, while tourism research has proceeded on the other, and for some unknown reason they have remained relatively isolated from one another."[37] However, an analysis of the *Journal of Travel Research* and the *Annals of Tourism Research* for the years 1977, 1980, 1983, and 1986 indicates that researchers affiliated with parks, recreation, and leisure are becoming more active in the area of tourism research.[38] In 1977 only 2.7 percent of the articles published in these two journals were authored by recreation researchers.[39] The proportion increased to 26.7 percent in 1986.[40]

Another area of increasing research interest is the relationship of tourism to the environment. Planners, landscape architects, and geographers have become more concerned about tourism's impact on the physical environment. A review of the literature on this relationship documents that "very few articles on the topic were in circulation during the mid-1960s and most on the subject have been published during the past 15 years."[41]

RESEARCH

Charles Goeldner, a prominent tourism researcher, has claimed that tourism researchers often fail to make effective use of secondary data.[42] Failure to thoroughly utilize existing data results in the time-consuming and costly collection of duplicative data. Secondary data frequently consist of descriptive studies that are based on surveys, questionnaires, interviews, and observation—all research techniques commonly used by social scientists. Using the comparative analysis of the *Journal of Travel Research* and the *Annals of Tourism Research* conducted by Richard R. Perdue, Ann A. Coughlin, and Laura Valerius in 1987 as a measure, the most frequently used research methods are survey research, the analysis of extant statistical data, and observation.[43]

Tourism researchers also make use of sophisticated mathematic models to simulate and predict tourist behavior. One example of an important model is the Travel Economic Impact Model developed by the U.S. Travel Data Center.[44] This computerized model estimates how much money travelers will spend in each state annually based on the estimates of spending in fourteen travel-related businesses. In order to develop a more comprehensive estimate of tourism's impact on state economies, the model also estimates the tax revenue, payroll income, and employment generated by tourism. This model is unique because it provides the only estimate of the economic impacts of travel in all fifty states and the District of Columbia.

Tourism researchers are becoming more interested in and also more experienced with the use of intricate methodologies. The Perdue, Coughlin, and Valerius study found that there was an increase in the number of articles published on tourism research methodologies from the late 1970s to the mid-1980s.[45] A study of the statistical methods used in articles published in the *Annals of Tourism Research*, the *Journal of Travel Research*, and *Tourism Management* for the period 1978-87 reported an increased use of complex as well as diverse research methods.[46] Statistics are a key component of scholarly tourism articles. Approximately 57 percent of the 659 articles analyzed made use of statistics.[47] Although descriptive statistics were most frequently used, more sophisticated techniques such as regression analysis, correlation, and modeling were also being used. The authors of the study concluded that tourism research is "moving slowly toward the advanced methodologies apparent in several well founded social science disciplines."[48]

DATA COLLECTION

The lack of uniform terminology in travel/tourism has already been examined. Tourism researchers, agencies, and organizations have persistently supported the need for standardization of definitions in order to make data comparable. Tourism also presents some other unique measurement problems. J. R. Brent Ritchie, a renowned tourism researcher, identified some of these specific complications in a seminal article published in 1975 in the *Journal of Travel Research*.[49] In fact this article is so significant that it has been reprinted in tourism textbooks as basic reading for students. Ritchie outlined variables that contribute to the collection of unreliable data. First, tourism data are often based on the willingness and ability of individuals to log or reconstruct the details of a trip such as the amount of money they spent on food, lodging, entertainment, sightseeing, and sourvenirs. Ritchie concluded that "while possible for one or several items, the complexity of travel expenditures makes total recall virtually impossible."[50] Also, travel/tourism is unlike other consumer purchases. It is generally not purchased on a regular basis and its luxury/exotic characteristic may lead to special problems in data collection. Because travel is often an escape from routine and reality, travelers are more likely to splurge. Consequently, tourism is not a typical consumer good. Tourism revenue is also hard to predict. Because pleasure travel is often viewed as nonessential, its consumption is affected by the purchase of other consumer durables such as cars and homes. In addition, some travel and tourism studies can never be replicated because they relate to unique events such as the Olympics. Ritchie later published an important article chronicling the difficulty of assessing the full impact of "hallmark events"[51] such as world fairs, Mardi Gras, the World Cup, royal weddings, and presidential inaugurations. Finally, tourism data are hard to collect because doing so involves an activity that is dispersed in terms of time and place. Travelers are hard to survey because they are on the go during a trip, and if they are surveyed too long after completing a trip, their recall may not be accurate.

Data collection in tourism research also presents other problems. The collection of data is costly and time consuming. This is partially due to the heavy use of survey research as a methodology. It is expensive to design questionnaires, to hire interviewers, and to collate and analyze the data. The process of collecting primary data generally involves at least several months of work. Unfortunately, data are often quickly out of date. Because tourism is a constantly changing activity, data have to be continuously collected. Cost and currency are also issues in data collection because many of the organizations involved in tourism research are relatively small in size and have limited resources.

Tourism data are being subjected to greater scrutiny. There have been charges that state governments have manipulated data and overestimated tourism revenue in order to receive more money for tourism development and promotion. Two researchers who recently conducted a detailed study on tourism methodology found that "tourism measurement is and remains an area plagued with inconsistency and ambiguity"[52] and suggested the need for "Regulation T ... Truth in Tourism Reporting."[53]

DATA PRODUCERS

Data on travel/tourism are often collected by the private sector. Companies who have a stake in the tourism industry may sponsor research. For example, the American Express Company collects data on business travelers and reports it in the *American Express Survey of Business Travel Management*. Airlines, hotels, motels, chain restaurants, and theme parks also collect data or pay consultants to gather information. Company-generated data tend to focus on marketing and feasibility studies. Because the data are paid for by corporations and are expensive to collect, companies may regard it as proprietary—that is, the results are not made available to the public.

Data are also collected by research centers such as the U.S. Travel Data Center, a not-for-profit research center. The Center is an excellent example of a cooperative effort by industry and government. The Center was organized in 1973 by the predecessor of the U.S. Travel and Tourism Administration and the Travel Industry Association of America. It is funded through membership fees, research contract fees, and money derived from the sale of publications. Its function is to conduct economic impact studies and market surveys.

Professional and trade associations are also important producers of tourism data. The Travel and Tourism Research Association, established in 1970, collects and disseminates travel and tourism data.[54] Its publications include the prestigious *Journal of Travel Research*. The association—whose membership includes airlines, hotels, motels, resorts, attractions, convention and visitors bureaus, government agencies, consultants, advertising agencies, and universities—also sponsors conferences, seminars, workshops, and meetings. Although the association is based in Salt Lake City, Utah, it operates the Travel Reference Center in Boulder, Colorado. This reference center is affiliated with the University of Colorado's Business Research Division and with more than 10,000 volumes represents the largest collection of tourism research material in this country. There is a separate fee structure for members and nonmembers of the Travel and Tourism Research Association.

Tourism data are also collected by government agencies. At the federal level in the United States, the U.S. Travel and Tourism Administration, part of the Department of Commerce, is the primary government agency responsible for tourism promotion. The goal of this agency in recent years has been the promotion of the United States as a destination for international visitors. State and local governments have also been active in promoting tourism. Each state has an office of tourism whose function is to develop and promote tourism in that state. Most large cities also have established convention and visitors bureaus to attract tourists.

Several international and intergovernmental agencies are involved in tourism research. The World Tourism Organization, based in Madrid, promotes tourism and acts as a clearinghouse for tourism information. Its members include national tourism organizations and trade associations. Along with conducting research and disseminating the results, it sponsors workshops and seminars. Two intergovernmental organizations that also produce tourism data are the Organization for Economic Cooperation and Development (OECD) and the Organization of American States (OAS). Outside the United

States, most countries have national tourist offices that collect statistics as well as promote tourism. They vary in name from country to country and may be called tourist boards, associations, or authorities.

USERS OF DATA

There are a myriad of tourism data users. All sectors of the tourism industry need information on which to base marketing decisions. The types of companies needing information on tourism include airlines, cruise lines, railroads, bus companies, tour operators, travel agents, attractions, hotels, motels, resorts, campgrounds, and recreational vehicle manufacturers. Consulting, advertising, and public relation agencies that work with these companies also need data. Government agencies at all levels are also interested in travel and tourism information. Finally, students and researchers at colleges and universities need to know how to access information relating to the tourism industry.

CHAPTER FOCUS

This chapter emphasizes sources leading to aggregate data on travel/tourism. Only selective sources on individual sectors of the tourism industry are included. For example, the role of consulting companies like Pannell Kerr Forster will be briefly discussed. This firm produces important statistical and trend data on the lodging industry. In addition, scholarly research sources are emphasized over popular consumer travel sources. The goal of the bibliography has been the identification and description of the bibliographies, monographs, dictionaries, encyclopedias, directories, indexes, databases, periodicals, proceedings, and statistical sources that constitute a core reference collection in tourism studies.

Tourism, like many social science disciplines, emphasizes current rather than retrospective works. Historical sources are not included unless they are classic works. Only English language materials have been selected for inclusion. Although much tourism literature is published in languages other than English, American researchers and students tend to rely exclusively on English-language material.

As has been documented earlier in this essay, tourism research is conducted across a number of social science disciplines. Tourism draws from geography, anthropology, economics, business, psychology, sociology, political science, law, leisure, and recreation. Readers needing background on social science research methodologies and a knowledge of basic sources in the social sciences should consult *The Social Sciences: A Cross-Disciplinary Guide to Selected Sources*, edited by Nancy L. Herron (Libraries Unlimited, 1989).

SOURCES

Guides and Handbooks

D-1. Ritchie, J. R. Brent, and Charles R. Goeldner, eds. **Travel, Tourism, and Hospitality Research: A Handbook for Managers and Researchers**. New York: Wiley, 1987.

Each of the forty-three chapters of this handbook can be read alone. It is assumed that chapters will be read selectively rather than consecutively. The editors have designed a book that can be used as a sourcebook for managers beginning research or as a textbook for students enrolled in tourism research courses. The roster of contributors is impressive. It includes leading tourism researchers in academe, industry, and tourism organizations. Some chapters address specific research methods. For example, there are chapters on the following methodologies: psychographics, enroute surveys, the delphi technique, nominal group techniques, and modeling. Other chapters are more theoretical and discuss the relationship of tourism to specific disciplines, definitional problems associated with tourism, and assessing the impacts of tourism.

Standard/Classic Sources

D-2. Feifer, Maxine. **Tourism in History: From Imperial Rome to the Present**. New York: Stein and Day, 1985.

This social history of tourism was first published in Great Britain under the title *Going Places*. The nine chapters explore tourism in different historical periods. Travel is seen through the eyes of the Imperial Roman, the medieval pilgrim, the Elizabethan, the Grand Tourist, the Romantic, the Victorian, the Belle Epoque Sojourner, the post-World War II mass tourist, and the contemporary American traveler. For each time period, Feifer develops a prototype of a tourist and creates a fictional account of what that tourist saw and did. These accounts are backed up by factual research, which Feifer cites in the bibliography that accompanies the text.

D-3. Gee, Chuck Y., James C. Makens, and Dexter J. L. Choy. **The Travel Industry**. 2d ed. New York: Van Nostrand Reinhold, 1989.

The second edition of this introductory text has expanded its coverage of the international dimension of tourism. The sixteen chapters are organized into six parts: overview of the travel industry, government role and public policy, tourism development, selling travel, transportation services, and hospitality and related services. Each chapter lays out objectives and identifies key terms. Discussion questions are included to reinforce concepts. This well-designed basic text covers all sectors of the tourism industry and has good coverage of current issues impacting the industry such as increased competition, deregulation, economic and political instability, and technological developments.

D-4. Gunn, Clare A. **Tourism Planning**. 2d ed. New York: Taylor & Francis, 1988.

Gunn, a professor emeritus of Texas A & M University's Recreation and Parks Department, is a widely respected authority on tourism design and planning. First published in 1979, this book established basic planning principles for tourism development and focused on the American experience. This revised edition has a more global perspective. There are numerous examples of tourism development in other countries and regions of the world. It remains the definitive text on tourism planning. Gunn is also the author of *Vacationscape: Designing Tourist Regions*, another influential book on tourism development.

D-5. Lundberg, Donald E. **The Tourist Business**. 6th ed. New York: Van Nostrand Reinhold, 1990.

This widely used text is in its sixth edition. It updates the material contained in the previous edition and has been strengthened by the addition of a chapter on travel geography, a primer on popular tourist destinations. After defining tourism, Lundberg traces its history and discusses why people travel. Subsequent chapters look at modes of transportation, accommodations, and the function of travel agencies. Other chapters look at destination marketing, destination development, and the social and economic impacts of tourism. There are also chapters on health problems encountered by travelers and the role of weather. The frequent use of concrete examples and practical advice have contributed to the popularity of this basic text.

D-6. MacCannell, Dean. **The Tourist: A New Theory of the Leisure Class**. New York: Schocken, 1976.

In 1973 MacCannell published an article on staged authenticity in an issue of the *American Journal of Sociology*. Staged authenticity refers to events that are contrived by hosts for the benefit and enjoyment of guests. This seminal article is reprinted here and MacCannell's views of the tourist are expanded. MacCannell's study combines a mixture of research methodologies, ranging from an analysis of Baedeker travel guides to personal observations based on extensive travels. This heavily cited work has become the standard sociological study of the modern middle class tourist.

D-7. McIntosh, Robert W., and Charles R. Goeldner. **Tourism: Principles, Practices, Philosophies**. 6th ed. New York: Wiley, 1989.

This standard textbook on tourism is now in its sixth edition. The authors have added a chapter on tourism as a force for world peace. Chapters cover the following: the definition and history of tourism; the organization and role of tourism organizations; the sectors composing the tourism industry; the economic, social, educational, and cultural aspects of tourism; tourism planning, development, and marketing; and travel and tourism research methods and sources of information. Both authors are recognized authorities. Their book is intended as an undergraduate level text as well as a primer for trade organizations, government agencies, and companies involved in researching, developing, or promoting tourism.

D-8. Mill, Robert Christie. **Tourism: The International Business**. Englewood Cliffs, NJ: Prentice-Hall, 1990.

This is Mill's second textbook on tourism. He previously coauthored *The Tourism System: An Introductory Text* with Alastair M. Morrison. *Tourism: The International Business* is also an undergraduate level text. The first section of the book provides an overview of tourism with chapters on the history of tourism, travel motivations, modes of transportation, tourist destinations, and tourism organizations. Part 2 focuses on the development, planning, and management of tourism. Part 3 covers tourism marketing. The final section addresses the future of tourism and discusses how tourism is affected by demographic and lifestyle changes. Review questions at the end of each chapter help to reinforce concepts. Three appendixes are provided: a brief bibliography, including a listing of major trade and professional associations; a glossary of terms; and a listing of major travel abbreviations. This readable and well-designed text is suitable for associate and baccalaureate level tourism curricula.

D-9.   Rosenow, John E., and Gerald L. Pulsipher. **Tourism: The Good, the Bad, and the Ugly**. Lincoln, NE: Century Three Press, 1979.

The authors use case studies to illustrate the positive and negative impacts of tourism in America. On the positive side, tourism can result in economic prosperity and the preservation of an area's natural beauty and historical heritage. On the negative side, tourism can result in a homogenization of culture as one town resembles another and can contribute to pollution, congestion, and other environmental problems. The authors promote planned tourism where local communities take actions to minimize the adverse impacts of tourism.

D-10.   Smith, Valene L., ed. **Hosts and Guests: The Anthropology of Tourism**. 2d ed. Philadelphia: University of Pennsylvania Press, 1989.

Although anthropologists have long recognized tourism's impact on indigenous cultures (the impact of guests on hosts), this volume, first published in 1977, was a pioneering work on the anthropology of tourism. The second edition updates the first by incorporating new research findings on the consequences of tourism. Through case studies, contributors examine tourism's role in both primitive and industrialized societies. Anthropology is often associated with the study of exotic cultures. Geographic regions selected for inclusion in this book range from Toraja in Indonesia to three coastal towns in North Carolina. Additional locales studied are Tonga, Bali, Polynesia, and Spain. Other populations analyzed are Eskimos, Iranian Jews, Indians of the American Southwest, and the Kuna Indians of Panama. An impressive bibliography comprises approximately fifty pages of the volume. This collection of fascinating case studies with thoughtful overview articles by Nelson H. H. Graburn, Dennison Nash, and Theron Nunez will remain basic reading on the cultural consequences of tourism.

D-11.   Stevens, Laurence. **Your Career in Travel, Tourism, and Hospitality**. 6th ed. Albany, NY: Delmar Publishers, 1988.

This title is part of the Travel Management Library Series published by Delmar. It is a revised edition of *Your Career in Travel and Tourism*. First issued in 1977, it has become a standard source for career information in the travel, tourism, and hospitality industries. The author is an authority, having managed a travel management consulting company since 1972. In addition, Stevens founded Merton House Travel & Tourism Publishers, a publishing house specializing in publications relating to travel agency management and travel and tourism. (Merton House became part of Delmar Publishers in 1986.) The first five chapters describe specific occupations, outlining responsibilities, qualifications, working conditions, and employment prospects. Chapter 6 covers fields relating to travel, tourism, and hospitality such as recreation and club management. The final chapter offers general advice on job hunting. This vocational guidance handbook should be on the shelves of high school, public, and academic libraries.

D-12.   Turner, Louis, and John Ash. **The Golden Hordes: International Tourism and the Pleasure Periphery**. New York: St. Martin's, 1976.

Turner and Ash regard mass tourists as rich, lazy barbarians. They are the "golden hordes." Tourism is viewed as a destructive force. This extremely pessimistic work has become a classic that is almost always cited in any literature reviewing the impacts of tourism.

Dissertations

D-13.   **Dissertation Abstracts International**. Ann Arbor, MI: University Microfilms, 1938- . Online and CD-ROM formats available.

Approximately 35,000 doctoral dissertations from more than 500 institutions are indexed annually in this source. Accompanying abstracts are author-prepared. The index is published in three separate parts: "Section A: The Humanities and Social Sciences"; "Section B: The Sciences and Engineering"; and "Section C: Worldwide." Dissertations are organized under broad categories that are subdivided. Two indexes are provided: author and keyword. Unfortunately, the keyword indexing approach often requires users to search under many terms in order to find dissertations on a given topic. The subject arrangement is also not always useful. For example, tourism is not a topic that is specific to any one academic subject. Dissertations relating to tourism can be found under many subjects, ranging from anthropology to urban and regional planning. The online and CD-ROM formats are often preferable to the printed index because they provide greater searching flexibility and are relatively easy to use. Most of the dissertations indexed in *Dissertation Abstracts International* may be purchased in print or microfilm format from University Microfilms International. (See entries A-37, B-19, and C-18.)

Bibliographies and Catalogs

D-14.   Engass, Peter. **Tourism and the Travel Industry: An Information Sourcebook**. Phoenix, AZ: Oryx, 1988.

This bibliography compiled by Peter Engass, a geography professor from Mount Holyoke College, is part of the Oryx Sourcebook Series in Business and Management. Engass lists and briefly describes almost 900 books, journals, newsletters, government publications, and conference proceedings relating to domestic and international travel and tourism. Annotations tend to be descriptive rather than critical. Business oriented materials are emphasized. This volume can be used as a supplement to Goeldner and Dicke's 1980 bibliography on travel, tourism, and recreation, *Bibliography of Tourism and Travel Research Studies, Reports and Articles*.

D-15.   Goeldner, C. R. **Data Sources for Tourism Research**. Boulder, CO: Business Research Division, Graduate School of Business Administration, University of Colorado, 1989.

This article-length document was published previously as chapter 15 in *Travel, Tourism, and Hospitality Research: A Handbook for Managers and Researchers* (entry D-1) under the title "Travel and Tourism Information Sources." Goeldner lists and in most cases describes basic sources that tourism researchers need to know about, including bibliographies, textbooks, literature review articles, statistical sources, periodicals, indexes, and databases. In addition to his experience as editor of the *Journal of Travel Research* (D-40), Goeldner coauthored a major bibliography on tourism with Karen Dicke. This nine-volume bibliography, entitled *Bibliography of Tourism and Travel Research Studies, Reports and Articles*, was published by the University of Colorado's Business Research Division in 1980. Goeldner and Dicke's bibliography is primarily useful for a retrospective review of the tourism literature because its coverage ends with sources published in 1980.

D-16.   Jafari, Jafar, et al. **Bibliographies on Tourism and Related Subjects: An Annotated Sourcebook**. Boulder, CO: Business Research Division, Graduate School of Business Administration, University of Colorado, 1988.

The compilers have listed and described 271 bibliographies on tourism, transportation, hospitality, recreation, and leisure. Although most items are bibliographies, a few review articles and books with significant bibliographies were selected for inclusion. Titles are arranged in alphabetical order. Access to information is enhanced through the author and subject indexes. Citations indicate useful information such as length of publication, price, and the publisher's address. Annotations are descriptive rather than evaluative. Almost all publications are English-language. However, a listing of the bibliographies published by France's Centre des Hautes Études Touristiques follows the annotations. A second edition is planned.

Dictionaries and Encyclopedias

D-17.   Metalka, Charles J., ed. **The Dictionary of Tourism**. 3d ed. Albany, NY: Delmar Publishers, 1990.

This A to Z dictionary defines contemporary terms that are frequently used in the tourism industry and in the academic study of tourism. Terminology and acronyms from all sectors of the industry are included. Because tourism has linkages to so many other disciplines, some of the terms relate to other fields such as economics, geography, and planning. The selective inclusion of organizations, associations, and governmental agencies is a particularly useful feature. Overall, definitions are clear and concise. This one-of-a-kind dictionary is a must for anyone who needs to understand the language used by travel agents, tour operators, cruise lines, airlines, railroads, meeting planners, hoteliers, restaurateurs, tourism researchers, and others involved in the activity or study of tourism.

Directories

D-18.   **Travel Industry Personnel Directory**. New York: Fairchild Books, 1988- . Annual.

This single-volume thumb-indexed directory with more than 20,000 listings is a bargain priced at $25. Although the title suggests that it is a listing of individuals only, it is in fact a comprehensive and current directory to all segments of the travel industry. It includes the names, addresses, telephone and fax numbers of domestic and international airlines, cruise lines, sightseeing tour uses, railroads, car rental agencies, hotels, tour operators, tourist information offices, travel organizations, state travel bureaus, government agencies, and special travel services ranging from currency exchanges to market research firms. This directory conveniently packages information that is contained in numerous specialized and more expensive directories. This is an indispensable ready-reference source for travel agents and other travel professionals, but it also belongs on the shelves of both public and academic libraries.

Indexes, Abstracts, and Databases

D-19. **ABI/Inform**. Louisville, KY: UMI Data Courier, 1971- . Weekly updates. Online and CD-ROM formats available.

This database indexes business oriented periodicals. References (with accompanying abstracts) are to articles in popular, trade, and scholarly journals. There is no print counterpart. Descriptors or subject headings relating to travel and tourism include "travel," "tourism," "travel industry," and "tours." This database also allows users to search under product codes. Several product codes relate to the travel and tourism industry. (See entry B-31.)

D-20. **Articles in Hospitality and Tourism**. Guildford, England: Library, University of Surrey, 1985- . Monthly.

Indexers from the libraries of Britain's University of Surrey, Oxford Polytechnic, and Dorset Institute examine more than 100 trade and scholarly journals monthly for articles relating to travel, tourism, foodservice, lodging, leisure, and recreation. Articles are indexed under one of more than 130 narrow subject headings within two broad categories: hospitality industry and tourism. Cross references direct users to related articles. One or two descriptive sentences accompany citations to indicate the subject of each article. This is the only specialized printed index in this field to be produced on a monthly rather than a quarterly basis. Although this index is produced in Europe, American libraries will find that there is good coverage of American topics. Libraries supporting tourism and/or hospitality programs will want to purchase it to supplement *The Hospitality Index* (entry D-24), *Leisure, Recreation and Tourism Abstracts* (entry D-25), *Lodging and Restaurant Index* (entry D-26), and the *Travel and Tourism Index* (entry D-33).

D-21. **Business Index**. Foster City, CA: Information Access Company, 1979- . Monthly, covering the two most recent years.

This index is produced in microfilm format. Like *Business Periodicals Index* (entries B-34 and D-22), it indexes a wide range of business oriented periodicals. While *Business Periodicals Index* scans approximately 300 popular, trade, and scholarly journals, *Business Index* scans more than 800. Although only a few journals (primarily trade) in tourism and hospitality are indexed, this is a good source for locating tourism articles in broader business periodicals.

D-22. **Business Periodicals Index**. New York: H. W. Wilson, 1958- . Monthly, except August, with bimonthly, semiannual, and annual cumulations. Online and CD-ROM formats available.

Popular, trade, and scholarly journals in all fields of business are indexed in this periodical index. Articles relating to travel and tourism can be found by searching the following subject headings: tourist trade, travel, business travel, vacations, air travel, automobile touring, ocean travel, cruise lines, travel agencies, travel agents, foreign visitors, package tours, convention bureaus, hotels and motels, resorts, restaurants, and amusement parks. "See" and "see also" references guide you to related subject headings. Corporate names may also be searched. This easy-to-use index is particularly good for locating travel and tourism articles in broader business publications. Although specialized travel and tourism periodicals are not indexed, a few hospitality journals have been selected for indexing such as *Hotel and Motel Management*, *Restaurant Business*, and *The Cornell Hotel and Restaurant Administration Quarterly* (entry D-35). (See entry B-34.)

D-23. **CAB Abstracts**. Wallingford, United Kingdom: CAB International, 1972- . Monthly updates.

This database contains a subfile labeled TOUR. TOUR is the computerized counterpart of *Leisure, Recreation and Tourism Abstracts* (entries A-55, C-47, and D-25). Like the printed source, the database contains references with informative abstracts of journal articles, books, government publications, and conference proceedings. Using the computerized version of this index allows a more powerful kind of searching. It enables you to create your own customized bibliography. You can establish your own parameters, such as language of publication, publication type, and date of publication.

D-24. **The Hospitality Index**. Washington, DC: Consortium of Hospitality Research Information Sources, 1988- . Quarterly.

Hospitality is the umbrella term for the business that encompasses the lodging, foodservice, travel and tourism industries. It involves a much broader spectrum of operations than just restaurants and hotels, including all travel and vacation-related enterprises from airline meals to casinos. Although there are many specialized periodicals in the area of travel and tourism, many additional articles can be found in related hospitality journals such as *Hotel and Motel Management, Hotels*, the *International Journal of Hospitality Management, Lodging*, and *Meetings and Conventions*. All these periodicals are indexed by subject in the *Hospitality Index*. The following travel and tourism journals are also indexed: the *Annals of Tourism Research* (entry D-34), *Journal of Travel Research* (entry D-40), *Tourism Management* (entry D-44), and *Travel and Tourism Analyst* (entry D-46). The index is a collaborative effort by a consortium of academic and industry specialists: the American Hotel and Motel Association, Cornell University's School of Hotel Administration, the University of Nevada — Las Vegas, and the University of Wisconsin — Stout. More than forty periodicals are indexed and articles are assigned an average of four different subject headings. Subject headings are based on the *American Hotel and Motel Association Thesaurus*, a listing of more than 1,600 descriptors. Entries are arranged alphabetically by subject heading and an asterisk is used to designate articles that indexers consider to be of special significance. A floppy disk version of the index, searchable through Inmagic software is also available.

D-25. **Leisure, Recreation and Tourism Abstracts**. Wallingford, United Kingdom: Commonwealth Agricultural Bureaux, 1976- . Quarterly. Available online.

Tourism and travel are two of the major subject areas included in this indexing and abstracting service. Separate author and subject indexes lead users to citations with substantive annotations. Although both English- and non-English-language journals are indexed, all abstracts are in English. Books, book chapters, conference proceedings, newsletters, research reports, theses, and other types of publications are also indexed. There is broad coverage of the world's literature on tourism given the wide ranging and large number of journals scanned for relevant articles. Some of the major tourism and hospitality journals indexed are: *Annals of Tourism Research* (entry D-34), the *Cornell Hotel and Restaurant Administration Quarterly* (entry D-35), *Hospitality Research Journal*, *International Journal of Hospitality Management*, *International Tourism Reports* (entry D-38), *Journal of Travel Research* (entry D-40), *Revue de Tourisme* (entry D-43), *Service Industries Journal*, *Tourism Management* (entry D-44), *Travel and Tourism Analyst* (entry D-46), and *Visions in Leisure and Business* (entry D-49). The records from this database may be searched online in a subset of the CAB Abstracts database (entry D-23). (See entry A-55 and C-47.)

D-26. **Lodging and Restaurant Index**. West Lafayette, IN: The Restaurant, Hotel, and Institutional Management Institute, 1987- . Quarterly.

This index is compiled by Judith M. Nixon, the librarian at Purdue University's School of Consumer and Family Sciences. It was first issued in 1985 as an in-house publication under the title *Index to Periodical Articles in the Restaurant, Hotel, Food Service and the Travel Industries*. More than forty journals are indexed by subject, including the *Annals of Tourism Research* (entry D-34), *Hospitality and Tourism Educator* (entry D-37), *Journal of Travel Research* (entry D-40), and *Tourism Management* (entry D-44). Articles are listed under alphabetically arranged subject headings. A thesaurus guides users to the appropriate subject headings as well as broader and more narrow terms that are searchable in the index. Like the *Hospitality Index* (entry D-24), this is a good source for locating travel and tourism articles that have been published in hospitality journals as well as in major travel and tourism periodicals. An electronic version using Inmagic or Searchmagic software is also available.

D-27. **PAIS International in Print**. New York: Public Affairs Information Service, 1991- . Monthly. Online and CD-ROM formats available.

PAIS International in Print replaces two long-established indexes: *PAIS Bulletin* and *PAIS Foreign Language Index*. This is an excellent index to use when researching issues with a political or economic orientation because the primary emphasis is public affairs. The subjects covered include: economics, law, political science, business, public administration, transportation, and international relations—all disciplines that relate to tourism. *PAIS* indexes not only periodicals but it also selectively indexes books, government publications, pamphlets, reports, and conference proceedings. There is good indexing of publications produced by the U.S. Travel Data Center and the World Tourism Organization. This source indexes material published in English, French, German, Portuguese, Italian, and Spanish. *PAIS* is just one of many social science indexes that can be used to retrieve articles on tourism. Some other useful indexes are: the *Social Sciences Index*, the *Social Sciences Citation Index* (see entry A-59), *Current Contents/Social and Behavioral Sciences*, *Abstracts in Anthropology*, and *Sociological Abstracts* (entry D-31). (See entry A-56.)

D-28. **Predicasts F and S Index Europe**. Cleveland, OH: Predicasts, 1978- . Monthly, with quarterly and annual cumulations. Available online.

This European edition of the *Predicasts F and S Index* covers business activities in Eastern and Western Europe. More than 750 business oriented publications are scanned for articles relating to mergers and acquisitions, new products, technological developments, and social and political events impacting company operations in Europe. Users can search for industry information in section 1, for country information in section 2, or for company information in section 3. *Predicasts F and S Index United*

States (entry D-30) and *Predicasts F and S Index International* (entry D-29) should be used to locate information on European company operations outside Europe.

D-29. **Predicasts F and S Index International**. Cleveland, OH: Predicasts, 1967- . Monthly, with quarterly and annual cumulations. Available online.

This international edition of the *Predicasts F and S Index* covers business activity in the following regions: Canada, Latin America, Africa, the Middle East, Asia, and Oceania. Industry information is organized under SIC codes in section 1. Industry and product information for regions and countries can be found in section 2. Company information can be found in section 3. Although the indexing is excellent, many users are frustrated by the lack of corresponding holdings in their library. Even major research libraries do not own a significant number of the periodicals indexed here. This is also a problem encountered with the European edition of this index.

D-30. **Predicasts F and S Index United States**. Cleveland, OH: Predicasts, 1960- . Weekly, with monthly, quarterly, and annual cumulations. Available online.

This index can be used to locate information on industries, products, and companies that has been published in almost 800 business oriented periodicals. The coverage of trade journals is exceptional. Unlike other periodical indexes, this one has no subject index per se. One can search the colored pages under SIC codes for industry information or search the white pages under company names. Many SIC codes represent the different components of the travel industry. The following are some of the SIC codes that should be searched in the colored pages for industry information: 40110(railroad passenger operations), 41400(bus charter services), 441200(passenger ships), 45100 (scheduled airlines), 47210(travel agents), 554100(gasoline stations), 556100(recreational vehicle dealers), 581200(eating places), 7010(lodging and tourist services), 70110(hotels and motels), 75100(motor vehicle rent and lease), 79490(outdoor recreation), 799600 (amusement parks), 7996100(theme parks), and 799900(recreation not elsewhere classified). Company names searchable in the white pages (American Airlines, American Express, Amtrak, Disney, Marriott, etc.) represent all sectors of the travel industry.

D-31. **Sociological Abstracts**. San Diego, CA: Sociological Abstracts, Inc., 1953- . 5 issues/yr. Online and CD-ROM formats available.

This is the major periodical index in the field of sociology. It also selectively indexes journals in related disciplines such as anthropology, political science, economics, education, and communications. The scope is international and all areas of sociology are covered. Two separate supplements index book reviews and conference papers. This index is particularly useful in locating literature on the social, cultural, historical, and economic aspects of tourism. (See entry A-60.)

D-32. **Trade and Industry Index**. Foster City, CA: Information Access Company, 1981- . Weekly updates.

This database corresponds in part to *Business Index* (entry D-21). More than 300 business and trade periodicals are comprehensively indexed and selectively abstracted. An additional 1,200 magazines and newspapers are scanned for industry related articles. *Trade and Industry ASAP*, a companion database, contains the full text of articles from more than 200 journals indexed in *Trade and Industry Index*. More than 100 local and regional business publications are included in *Area Business Databank*, a subfile of *Trade and Industry Index*. *Trade and Industry Index* also contains news releases that have been prepared by companies, trade associations, government agencies, and other sources. All types of industries are represented in this database and the inclusion of business, trade-specific, and nonbusiness periodicals results in a wide range of articles on any given topic. For example, a quick search on the impact of terrorism on tourism retrieved citations ranging from the *Travel Agent* to the *Public Relations Journal*.

D-33. **Travel and Tourism Index**. Laie, HI: Brigham Young University, Hawaii Campus, 1984- . Quarterly.

This is a subject index to travel and tourism articles published in consumer travel magazines, newsletters, trade periodicals, and scholarly journals. Forty-five periodicals are indexed, including many that are not indexed elsewhere. It has particularly good coverage of articles relating to the Pacific Rim region—the huge geographic area encompassing the countries, islands, and regions surrounded by the Pacific Ocean. This West Coast and Asian emphasis (no doubt influenced by the index's Hawaiian base) is illustrated by the indexing of periodicals such as *Business Traveller* (Asia/ Pacific Edition), *China Tourism*, *PATA Travel News* (Asia/Pacific), and *Travelage West*. Although the journals selected for indexing are diverse, this index is by no means comprehensive and it should not be relied on exclusively to locate articles relating to travel and tourism. For example, two major scholarly journals are excluded from indexing: *International Tourism Reports* (entry D-38) and *Travel and Tourism Analyst* (entry D-46). Nevertheless, it is a good companion to other indexes that include research on travel and tourism.

Core Journals

D-34. **Annals of Tourism Research: A Social Sciences Journal**. New York: Pergamon, 1974- . Quarterly.

This academic journal regards tourism as a social science. Articles are contributed by scholars from a broad range of disciplines: geography, anthropology, economics, leisure and recreation, planning, public administration, political science, history, business administration, psychology, and sociology. Special issues of the journal have examined tourism's relationship to other disciplines. Volumes have been devoted to the following themes: the sociology of tourism; the geography of tourism; the anthropology of tourism; political science and tourism; and the linkage between leisure, recreation, and tourism. In addition to publishing substantial research articles, there are conference reports, research reports, book reviews, and a listing of recent publications. This journal is indexed in *Articles in Hospitality and Tourism* (entry D-20), *Hospitality Index* (entry D-24), *Lodging and Restaurant Index* (entry D-26), *Leisure, Recreation and Tourism Abstracts* (entry D-25), *Travel and Tourism Index* (entry D-33), and *Touristic Analysis Review* (entry D-45). It is also indexed in several broad social science indexes.

D-35. **Cornell Hotel and Restaurant Administration Quarterly**. Ithaca, NY: School of Hotel Administration, 1960- . Quarterly.

This prestigious journal is published by Cornell University's School of Hotel Administration, the premier hospitality education program in this country. It is indexed in *ABI/Inform* (entry D-19), *Articles in Hospitality and Tourism* (entry D-20), *Business Index* (entry D-21), *Business Periodicals Index* (entry D-22), the *Hospitality Index* (entry D-24), *Leisure, Recreation and Tourism Abstracts* (entry D-25), *Lodging and Restaurant Index* (entry D-26), *Touristic Analysis Review* (entry D-45), and *Trade and Industry Index* (entry D-32). Research articles cover the restaurant, lodging, and travel industries and focus on management concerns. This journal is also a good source of current industry news. The August issues features the "Educator's Forum," a special annual issue on hospitality education.

D-36.   **From the State Capitals. Tourist Business Promotion**. New Haven, CT: Wakeman/Walworth, 1982- . Monthly.

This is one of the newsletters published by Wakeman/Walworth in their From the State Capitals series. In eight pages it provides news about state and municipal efforts to promote tourism. State tourist offices, visitor and convention bureaus, and local chambers of commerce may find some useful ideas in this unique newsletter, which is not covered by any indexing service.

D-37.   **Hospitality and Tourism Educator**. Washington, DC: Council on Hotel, Restaurant and Institutional Education, 1988- . 3 issues/yr.

This journal is published by the Council on Hotel, Restaurant and Institutional Education (CHRIE), the primary organization for hospitality and tourism educators. CHRIE was founded in 1946 and includes more than 1,400 members from academia and industry. Each issue of *Hospitality and Tourism Educator* publishes articles of interest both to educators and to industry recruiters because the goal of the journal is to bridge education and industry. This journal is indexed in the *Lodging and Restaurant Index* (entry D-26). CHRIE also publishes *Hospitality Research Journal* (formerly *Hospitality Education and Research Journal*), the leading research journal in hospitality education.

D-38.   **International Tourism Reports**. London: Economist Intelligence Unit, 1971- . Quarterly.

Each issue contains detailed reports on individual tourism markets. Well established markets are covered, but there are also reports on small markets that demonstrate a potential for growth. Each report traces the development of tourism in a nation or region, analyzes trends, and provides extensive statistical data on such things as tourist arrivals, tourism receipts, and accommodations. The scope is global, covering Algeria to Zimbabwe. This is an indispensable source to tourism researchers, marketers, and planners needing an analysis of international markets. This journal is indexed in *Articles in Hospitality and Tourism* (entry D-20) and *Leisure, Recreation and Tourism Abstracts* (entry D-25).

D-39.   **Journal of Leisure Research**. Alexandria, VA: National Recreation and Park Association, 1968- . Quarterly. Indexed in *Leisure, Recreation and Tourism Abstracts*.

This scholarly journal is published by the National Recreation and Park Association in cooperation with the University of North Texas. It publishes a wide range of research articles relating to leisure and recreation. Many of them, such as the article on vacation satisfaction, are relevant to tourism research. Its importance as a source of tourism data is reflected by its indexing in *Articles in Hospitality and Tourism* (entry D-20), *Hospitality Index* (D-24), and the *Lodging and Restaurant Index* (entry D-26). (See entry A-63.)

D-40. **Journal of Travel Research**. Boulder, CO: Business Research Division, Graduate School of Business Administration, University of Colorado, 1962- . Quarterly.

This journal is published by the Travel and Tourism Research Association, a professional association whose members include representatives from academia, industry, and government. Its research articles address issues in all sectors of the tourism industry and are contributed by academic researchers and industry specialists. The journal also includes a section containing conference reports and shorter articles reporting on pilot studies. "Travel Research Bookshelf," an annotated bibliography of recent books, reports, and journal articles, is a regular feature. There are also longer reviews of two or three books in each issue. It is indexed in *ABI/Inform* (entry D-19), *Articles in Hospitality and Tourism* (entry D-20), *Business Periodicals Index* (entry D-22), *The Hospitality Index* (entry D-24), *Leisure, Recreation and Tourism Abstracts* (entry D-25), *Lodging and Restaurant Index* (entry D-26), *Touristic Analysis Review* (entry D-45), and *Travel and Tourism Index* (entry D-33). *The Journal of Travel Research* (entry D-40) and *Annals of Tourism Research* (entry D-34) are the two leading journals in tourism studies and are basic to any academic program in travel and tourism.

D-41. **Leisure Sciences**. New York: Taylor & Francis, 1977- . Quarterly.

This scholarly journal approaches leisure from an interdisciplinary perspective. Articles tend to be theoretical rather than applied. Tourism-related articles often focus on methodologies, such as modeling systems. Lengthy book reviews are included as well as a calendar of upcoming meetings and conferences. This journal is indexed in *Articles in Hospitality and Tourism* (entry D-20), *Leisure, Recreation and Tourism Abstracts* (entry D-25), *Touristic Analysis Review* (entry D-45), and several social science indexes. (See entry A-68.)

D-42. **Progress in Tourism, Recreation and Hospitality Management**. London: Belhaven Press, 1989- . Annual.

Each volume publishes several review articles as well as shorter articles on advances in tourism, recreation, and hospitality management. This is the first periodical that fully integrates these three disciplines. It also effectively brings together both theoretical and applied research. It is indexed in *Articles in Hospitality and Tourism* (entry D-20) and *Leisure, Recreation and Tourism Abstracts* (entry D-25).

D-43. **Revue de Tourisme/The Tourist Review/Zeitschrift für Fremdenverkehr**. Bern, Switzerland: Association Internationale d'Experts Scientifiques du Tourisme (AIEST), 1946- . Quarterly.

This long-established research journal in tourism publishes articles in English, French, and German. English-language abstracts are provided for articles published in French or German. A calendar section lists notices of future conferences and highlights of recently held conferences. There is also a listing of books received and a small number of book reviews. It is indexed in *Articles in Hospitality and Tourism* (entry D-20), *Leisure, Recreation and Tourism Abstracts* (entry D-25), and the *Travel and Tourism Index* (entry D-33). This is the official publication of AIEST, an association of tourism researchers and educators. The association also publishes the proceedings of its annual conference.

D-44. **Tourism Management**. Guildford, England: Butterworth Scientific, 1980- . Quarterly.

Although this international journal emerged only a decade ago, it is regarded as one of the leading scholarly journals in the field. The focus is on tourism planning and development. There are short articles on current issues and thought-provoking editorials. For example, a recent editorial debated whether or not tourism is a force for peace. In addition, there are long research articles, reports of projects in development, and book reviews. This journal is indexed in several sources, including *Articles in Hospitality and Tourism* (entry D-20), *Hospitality Index* (entry D-24), *Leisure, Recreation and Tourism Abstracts* (entry D-25), *Lodging and Restaurant Index* (entry D-26), and *Touristic Analysis Review* (entry D-45).

D-45. **Touristic Analysis Review**. Aix-en-Provence, France: Centre des Hautes Études Touristiques, 1973- . Quarterly.

The Centre is affiliated with Aix-en-Provence University, the sole university in France to offer a doctoral degree in tourism. The Centre has an extensive collection of tourism publications. This English-language journal lists and describes recent books, book chapters, and scholarly articles relating to tourism. It can be used by researchers as a current awareness service and by librarians as a collection development aid. The following journals are scanned for tourism articles: *Annals of Tourism Research* (entry D-34), *Journal of Travel Research* (entry D-40), *International Tourism Reports* (entry D-38), *Tourism Management* (entry D-44), *Travel and Tourism Analyst* (entry D-46), *Visions in Leisure and Business* (entry D-49), *International Journal of Hospitality Management*, the *Cornell Hotel and Restaurant Administration Quarterly* (entry D-35), *Leisure Studies*, *Leisure Sciences* (entry D-41), the *Journal of Park and Recreation Administration*, and the *Service Industries Journal*. The addition of author and subject indexes would greatly improve this otherwise excellent source.

D-46. **Travel and Tourism Analyst**. London: Economist Intelligence Unit, 1986- . Monthly.

Each issue contains in-depth research reports on different sectors of the tourism industry. These reports gather data from published and unpublished sources. While *International Tourism Reports* (see entry D-38), another Economist publication, reports on individual country markets, *Travel and Tourism Analyst* analyzes and forecasts broader industry trends. For example, there have been reports on the Mediterranean cruise industry, the car rental industry in the United States, and major hotel chains operating in Asia. Like many Economist publications, this journal is very expensive. It collects and interprets fragmented and hard-to-find data as a service to industry practitioners. Although planners and analysts from all sectors of the tourism industry subscribe to it, it is likely to be found only in major research libraries. It is indexed in *Articles in Hospitality and Tourism* (entry D-20), *The Hospitality Index* (entry D-24), *Leisure, Recreation and Tourism Abstracts* (entry D-25), and *Touristic Analysis Review* (entry D-45).

D-47. **Travel Printout: Research News from the U.S. Travel Data Center**. Washington, DC: U.S. Travel Data Center, 1972- . Monthly.

This monthly four- to six-page newsletter reports tourism data for the previous two to five months. Summary data from the following statistical series are regularly featured: the Travel Price Index, Current Travel Indicators, the National Travel Survey, and Visitor Volume at National Parks. Data are derived from the U.S. Travel Data Center and other public and private sources such as the U.S. Bureau of Labor

Statistics, the U.S. Travel and Tourism Administration, the Federal Highway Administration, the National Park Service, the U.S. Department of Energy, Amtrak, the Air
Transport Association, Smith Travel Research, and the Conference Board. Articles
from industry experts and commentary by the Center's executive director are also
regular features. In addition, there are conference reports and news about the Center's
activities. This is a good current awareness source for individuals and organizations
researching the U.S. travel industry. It is indexed in the *Statistical Reference Index*
(entry D-55) and the *Travel and Tourism Index* (entry D-33).

D-48. **Travel Weekly**. Secaucus, NJ: Murdoch Magazines, 1958- . Semiweekly.

This semiweekly newspaper is subtitled "the national newspaper of the travel
industry." It is a good source of current information on fares, booking patterns,
government regulations, mergers and acquisitions, and personnel changes. Each issue
of this glossy, oversized periodical contains numerous advertisements for cruise lines,
hotels, car rental agencies, airlines, and other travel-related services. There is also a
section listing job opportunities. This is read regularly by travel agents and other
persons involved in travel marketing and sales. It is indexed in *Business Index* (entry
D-21), *Travel and Tourism Index* (entry D-33), and *Trade and Industry Index* (entry
D-32).

D-49. **Visions in Leisure and Business**. Bowling Green, OH: Appalachian Associates,
1982- . Quarterly.

This journal was launched in 1982 with the purpose of filling a perceived gap
between the applied leisure sciences and business. The editorial board consists of a good
balance of academicians and industry practitioners. Articles contain both theoretical
and practical information about the leisure service industries. There have been travel
and tourism articles on the seasonality of tourism, the senior travel market, problems of
tourism methodology, the costs and benefits of seasonal tourism to municipal governments, and tourism in the Bahamas. This journal is indexed in *Articles in Hospitality
and Tourism* (entry D-20), *Leisure, Recreation and Tourism Abstracts* (entry D-25),
and *Touristic Analysis Review* (entry D-45).

Conference Proceedings

D-50. **Outlook for Travel and Tourism: Proceedings of the ... Annual Travel Outlook
Forum**. Washington, DC: U.S. Travel Data Center, 1978- . Annual.

This annual conference is jointly sponsored by the U.S. Travel Data Center and
the Travel and Tourism Research Association. This collection of consistently excellent
papers delivered by industry specialists is a rich source of statistical and projective data.
Speakers representing all sectors of the industry address both the dilemmas and opportunities facing the tourism industry. Many participants suggest marketing strategies that
can be used to capitalize on demographic and economic trends. This is an important
source of information for state tourism offices, convention and visitors bureaus, and
businesses involved in travel-related marketing and sales.

D-51. Travel and Tourism Research Association. **Proceedings of the Annual Conference**. Salt Lake City, UT: Bureau of Economic and Business Research, Graduate School of Business, University of Utah, 1970- . Annual.

The Travel and Tourism Research Association (TTRA), formerly The Travel Research Association, was founded in 1970. It is an international association of travel researchers, marketers, planners, and developers. The TTRA annual conference assembles travel and tourism leaders from industry, government, and academia. Each conference has a unique theme. Some past themes are: Travel Research Globalization— The Pacific Rim and Beyond (1989); Tourism Research: Expanding Boundaries (1988); Travel and Tourism: Thrive or Survive (1987); Technology and Tourism: A Growing Partnership (1986); The Battle for Market Share: Strategies in Research and Marketing (1985); Travel Research: The Catalyst for Worldwide Tourism Marketing (1984); and Travel Research: Its Impact on the Travel Marketing Process (1983). These proceedings will be of interest to individuals and organizations involved in travel research and marketing.

D-52. U.S. Travel and Tourism Administration and the Travel and Tourism Research Association. **Proceedings of the Annual Travel Review Conference of the U.S. Travel and Tourism Administration and the Travel and Tourism Research Association.** Salt Lake City, UT: Travel and Tourism Research Association (TTRA), 1987- . Annual.

Government and industry specialists have gathered annually since 1987 to review the performance of the travel industry and to assess the outlook for the future. Conference speakers have included representatives from the following agencies: the U.S. Travel Data Center, the U.S. Travel and Tourism Administration, the Department of Transportation, the National Park Service, and Tourism Canada. Trade associations are also well represented. There have been participants from the following associations: the American Automobile Association, the United States Tour Operators Association, the American Hotel and Motel Association, the Professional Association of Innkeepers International, the American Association of Retired Persons, the International Association of Convention and Visitors Bureaus, the American Society of Travel Agents, the Cruise Lines International Association, the Travel and Tourism Research Association, and the International Association of Amusement Parks and Attractions. Some addresses have been delivered by industry consultants and by company representatives from, for example, National Car Rental, Amtrak, USAir, Carnival Cruise Lines, and Hilton Hotels. Most of the papers are enhanced by graphic depictions of statistical data. These proceedings are required reading for anyone involved in tourism planning and marketing.

Statistical Indexes

D-53. **American Statistics Index**. Bethesda, MD: Congressional Information Service, 1973- . Monthly, with annual cumulations. Online and CD-ROM formats available.

This source indexes statistical data found in publications of the federal government. There is an index volume and an abstracts volume. A corresponding microfiche collection is also available. This superb index provides detailed access to the vast number of statistical publications that are produced by all agencies and branches of the federal government. These publications are valuable sources of economic, demographic, and marketing data. Tourism researchers will also want to become familiar with this source because it indexes the publications of the U.S. Travel and Tourism Administration. (See entries A-79 and C-77.)

D-54. **Index to International Statistics**. Bethesda, MD: Congressional Information Service, 1983- . Monthly, with annual cumulations. CD-ROM format available.

This index is a companion to the *American Statistics Index* (entry D-53) and the *Statistical Reference Index* (entry D-55). It indexes English-language statistics that are found in the publications of international intergovernmental agencies. There is a corresponding microfiche collection. This is valuable to tourism researchers because it indexes the publications of the World Tourism Organization, the Organization for European Cooperation and Development, and the Organization of American States.

D-55. **Statistical Reference Index**. Bethesda, MD: Congressional Information Service, 1980- . Monthly, with annual cumulations. CD-ROM format available.

While the *American Statistics Index* (entry D-53) indexes federal publications, this source indexes statistical publications produced by state governmental agencies. In addition, it indexes statistical data found in the publications of private organizations. These include the publications issued by associations, business organizations, commercial publishers, and independent research organizations. This is a critical source for tourism researchers because it indexes statistics found in the publications of the U.S. Travel Data Center.

Statistical Sources

D-56. **The American Express Survey of Business Travel Management**. New York: American Express Travel Related Services, 1986- . Biennial.

This is the only comprehensive survey of American corporate travel policies. Data are based on a survey of almost 1,600 American businesses with at least 100 employees. Businesses surveyed include public and private companies, governmental agencies, and educational institutions. The survey covers the following items: travel patterns and costs, travel policies, travel arrangements, use of payment methods, and expense reporting and reconciliation. Because corporations have a continuous need to contain travel costs, this volume is a big seller, even at the price of $190. Travel managers and executives will find the money well spent.

D-57. Bar-On, Ray. **Travel and Tourism Data: A Comprehensive Research Handbook on the World Travel Industry**. Phoenix, AZ: Oryx, 1989.

The title of this book is somewhat misleading. This is not a general guide to sources of information for the study of travel and tourism. Almost half of this book consists of statistical data on tourism in more than 200 countries for the period 1982 to 1986. Other chapters focus on definitions of travel and tourism, sources of data, and methods of collecting and classifying data, including a separate chapter on analyzing and forecasting time series data. The author's inclusion of public data sources for individual countries is a particularly useful feature. This volume is intended for specialists. It was published simultaneously in Britain by Euromonitor.

D-58. **Compendium of Tourism Statistics**. Madrid: World Tourism Organization, 1975- . Annual.

This statistical abstract provides tourism data and basic economic data, such as area and population figures, for more than 180 countries and territories. Data generally cover a five-year time period. Most of the data are from the World Tourism Organization's annual *Yearbook of Tourism Statistics* (entry D-76) and its quarterly *Current Travel and Tourism Indicators*. Demographic and economic data are drawn from publications issued by the United Nations, the World Bank, and the International Monetary Fund. This compendium serves as a ready-reference guide on tourism in individual countries. The *Yearbook of Tourism Statistics* (entry D-76) can be used to answer questions requiring greater detail.

D-59. **The Economic Review of Travel in America**. Washington, DC: U.S. Travel Data Center, 1980- . Annual.

This annual report reviews the role of travel and tourism in the U.S. economy. It focuses on the past year, but data from previous years are included to allow comparison. There are statistics on travel spending, travel industry receipts, travel prices, and travel-generated employment. This information is used to determine industry trends and to assess travel and tourism's direct contribution to the overall U.S. economy. The Center provides summaries and interpretations of the data. Well-written narrative is enhanced by excellent graphics. This source is essential to anyone documenting the importance of tourism as an economic activity.

D-60. Edwards, Anthony. **International Tourism Forecasts to 1995**. London: The Economist Publications, 1985.

International Tourism Reports (entry D-38) and *Travel and Tourism Analyst* (entry D-46) are the quarterly and monthly publications of the Economist Intelligence Unit (EIU). Topics that warrant longer analyses than can be accommodated in these journals are the subjects of EIU Special Reports. *International Tourism Forecasts to 1995* is one of these special reports. Edwards forecasts the growth of international tourism from twenty main origin countries—the twenty top spenders. These countries are: Australia, Austria, Belgium, Canada, Denmark, France, West Germany, Italy, Japan, Kuwait, Mexico, Netherlands, Norway, Saudi Arabia, Spain, Sweden, Switzerland, the United Kingdom, the United States, and Venezuela. Projections are based on a sophisticated methodology that analyzes trends for the period from 1967 to 1982. This base study was updated by Edwards with the publication of *International Tourism Forecasts to 1999* (The Economist Intelligence Unit, 1988).

D-61. **European Travel Trends and Prospects, 1980-1995**. London: Euromonitor, 1988.

Although Euromonitor conducted research for this report, many of its estimates of tourism growth are based on secondary data, primarily statistics collected by the World Tourism Organization and the Organization for Economic Cooperation and Development. The report focuses on current trends and prospects for the future, but it also provides some historical background about the development of tourism in Europe. There are statistics pertaining to tourism in individual countries as well as aggregate data on European and world travel.

D-62. **The Impact of Travel on State Economies**. Washington, DC: U.S. Travel Data Center, 1974- . Annual.

The Travel Economic Impact Model (TEIM) is a computerized economic model that was developed by the U.S. Travel Data Center to estimate the economic impact of domestic travel in each U.S. state. The model measures expenditures, employment, payroll income, business receipts, and tax revenues generated by travel. Data are shown in detail. For example, travel spending is estimated in six categories: public transportation, auto transportation, lodging, foodservice, entertainment and recreation, and general retail trade. The data contained in the *Impact of Travel on State Economies* are unique. It is the only source to provide an estimate of the economic impact of travel for each of the fifty states and the District of Columbia. This is an essential source for state tourist offices and for analysts from all sectors of the tourism industry.

D-63. **Survey of Business Travelers**. Washington, DC: U.S. Travel Data Center, 1987- . Annual.

Almost 4,000 business travelers are interviewed by telephone during the year. Business travelers are defined as individuals who have traveled 100 miles or more one way for business or convention purposes during the past twelve months. They are asked about their reasons for traveling, how they selected hotels, the type of transportation they used, their use of travel agents, and whether they combined business and vacation. There are detailed demographic data about segments of business travelers such as, women, travelers aged 35-44, and travelers who travel to attend meetings. The thorough analysis of this significant segment of the overall travel market will be of particular interest to meeting planners, travel agents, car rental agencies, hotels, and airlines.

D-64. **Survey of State Travel Offices**. Washington, DC: U.S. Travel Data Center, 1973- . Annual.

State travel offices vary in size from fewer than 5 to more than 100 full-time employees. Their location within state governments also differs. Although some travel offices are organized as independent agencies that report directly to the governor, most offices are part of another department or agency such as commerce, economic development, parks, recreation, or community affairs. Projected 1989-90 state travel office budgets ranged from $1 million to more than $22 million. Comparison between states is made possible through the publication of the *Survey of State Travel Offices*, the results of a survey that has been conducted annually by the U.S. Travel Data Center since 1973. Data contained in the report are based on a questionnaire sent to the travel office in all fifty states, the District of Columbia, American Samoa, and Guam. Offices are asked to provide information about the following: general administration, advertising, budget, general promotion of tourism, package tours, press and public relations, research, and welcome centers. Responses are collated and presented in detailed tables; a summary and analysis are provided by the U.S. Travel Data Center. This comparative statistical compilation will be useful to government agencies, tourism researchers, travel organizations, and travel-related businesses.

D-65. **Tourism Policy and International Tourism in OECD Member Countries**. Paris: Organization for Economic Cooperation and Development, 1953- . Annual.

This statistical series studies the evolution of the tourist trade in the twenty-four OECD member countries. These twenty-four nations are: Australia, Austria, Belgium, Canada, Denmark, Finland, France, Germany, Greece, Iceland, Ireland, Italy, Japan, Luxembourg, the Netherlands, New Zealand, Norway, Portugal, Sweden, Switzerland, Turkey, the United Kingdom, the United States, and Yugoslavia. Data are shown in great detail. It is possible to find the following information for individual countries:

employment in the tourism industry (with a breakdown by sex), length of stay by foreign tourists, nights spent by foreign and domestic tourists by type of accommodation, foreign tourism by trip purpose, and tourism receipts and expenditures. This report documents the importance of international tourism as an economic activity, including data demonstrating the economic importance of travel in the balance of payments. It also provides information on governmental policies relating to tourism in individual OECD countries. In addition, it reports transportation policies that impact tourist movements by automobile, rail, air, or ship. This is a key source of statistical data on tourism in OECD countries.

D-66. **Tourism's Top Twenty: Fast Facts on Travel and Tourism**. 1988 ed. Boulder, CO: Business Research Division, Graduate School of Business Administration, University of Colorado; Washington, DC: U.S. Travel Data Center, 1987.

What is the world's busiest airport? What state has the highest percentage of travel-generated employment? What national park gets the most visitors? The answers to these questions can be found in *Tourism's Top Twenty*, a compendium of frequently requested figures relating to travel and tourism. The statistics cover all sectors of the travel and tourism industry: transportation, accommodations, attractions, foodservice, recreation, and sports. Although the data relate primarily to the United States, there are also statistics on world tourism. Data are presented in tabular form. The source of the data is clearly identified at the foot of each table. Sources for data include government agencies, trade associations, research centers, consultants, and commercial and trade publishers. There is also a subject index that enhances access to the data contained in the 101 tables. This handy statistical is usually updated every four years.

D-67. **Travel and Leisure's World Travel Overview: The Annual Review of the Travel Industry Worldwide**. New York: American Express Publishing Corp., 1986- . Annual.

This annual review of travel trends and travel markets is produced by *Travel and Leisure* in conjunction with the American Express Publishing Corporation. *Travel and Leisure* is a popular consumer travel magazine, but this report is directed to industry specialists. Like the *Travel Industry World Yearbook* (entry D-69), this is a compilation of industry statistics derived from associations, consultants, government agencies, and trade publishers. However, this publication is unique because of its five-year projections. *Travel and Leisure* has developed an exclusive model, Travel and Leisure's Travel Analysis Model (TRAM), to forecast travel to specific international markets. This is an essential source for industry executives involved in long-term planning.

D-68. **Travel Executive Briefing: A National Travel Survey Summary**. Washington, DC: U.S. Travel Data Center, 1987- . Quarterly.

These reports analyze seasonal travel. The source of the data is the Center's National Travel Survey, a monthly telephone survey of a national probability sample of 1,500 U.S. residents. Statistics are measured for winter, spring, summer, and autumn with comparisons to the same season of the previous year or to seasonal trends. The report analyzes travel demographics (marital status, sex, age, education, and family income); trip purposes (vacation, pleasure, business/convention, or weekend); and trip characteristics (such as primary transport mode, travel party size, traveling with or without children, lodging used, destination, and trip duration). There are also statistics showing travel prices and data on the overall U.S. economy. Reports are released in a timely fashion, generally within twelve weeks of a season's end. Similar data are reported annually in another Center publication, *Travel Executive Briefing: A National Travel Survey Summary*.

D-69.   **Travel Industry World Yearbook: The Big Picture**. New York: Child & Waters, 1956- . Annual.

Somerset R. Waters, a preeminent travel researcher and one of the founders of the Travel Research Association, has been the compiler of this statistical sourcebook for almost twenty years. Data are drawn from a variety of public and private sources: the World Tourism Administration, the U.S. Travel Data Center, the U.S. Travel and Tourism Administration, the Organization for Economic Cooperation and Development, the U.S. Department of Commerce, Pannell Kerr Forster, Ogilvy & Mather, Statistics Canada, the Caribbean Tourism Research and Development Centre, and the Pacific Asia Travel Association. Some data are produced by Child & Waters. This book is more than a collection of statistics. The data are interpreted and used as the basis for projecting tourism trends. World tourism trends and important political and economic events of the year are reviewed. There is an analysis of tourism in individual countries, in each U.S. state, and by sectors of the tourism industry (lodging, transportation, travel agencies, tour operators, and foodservice). This annual digest conveniently assembles and reviews critical data, providing a valuable service to individuals involved in tourism research or marketing of travel-related services.

D-70.   **Travel Market Close-Up: National Travel Survey Tabulations**. Washington, DC: U.S. Travel Data Center, 1987- . Quarterly.

This quarterly publication is a companion to *Executive Briefing: A National Travel Survey Summary*. It presents detailed seasonal data on various segments of the U.S. travel market. For example, there are profiles of weekend, business, senior, and affluent travelers. Data are based on the Center's National Travel Survey. *Travel Market Close-Up* is published within three months of the end of each season and it is a valuable source for tourism researchers and marketers. The Center also publishes *Travel Market Close-Up: National Travel Survey Tabulations*, an annual report providing similar data.

D-71.   **Travel Trends in the United States and Canada**. Boulder, CO: Business Research Division, Graduate School of Business Administration, University of Colorado, 1960- . Irregular.

More than 250 sources were consulted for the preparation of the 1984 edition. Data were collected through 1982 for U.S. states and Canadian provinces. In some cases, data were projected beyond 1982. Many of the 108 tables contain statistical series going back to 1970. Although statistics are not current, this is still a good source of historical data on tourist expenditures, travel-generated employment, tourism advertising, travel costs, passport statistics, tourist visits, visits to recreational areas, and the economic impact of tourism.

D-72.   **Trends in the Hotel Industry, International Edition**. New York: Pannell Kerr Forster, 1981- . Annual.

This annual publication reports on the operating results of the non-U.S. hotel industry. More than 500 worldwide hotels and 1,000 U.S. hotels are surveyed. The report compares the performance of international hotels to U.S. hotels. Data are summarized for regions and countries. The following regions are covered: Latin

America, the Caribbean, Europe, the Middle East, Africa, the Pacific Basin, Canada, and Mexico. Comparisons are made to the previous year. Trend data are also reported.

D-73. **Trends in the Hotel Industry, USA Edition**. New York: Pannell Kerr Forster, 1980- . Annual.

This annual review of hotel operations in the United States is based on Pannell Kerr Forster's survey of 1,000 hotels and motels. Although the focus is on the financial performance of the industry during the past year, there is comparison to the year before as well as a summary of the trends for the past twenty years. There is also projective data for the forthcoming year. The analysis of hotel performance by region, state, and city is particularly useful to hoteliers, meeting planners, visitor and convention bureaus, and state travel offices.

D-74. **U.S. Lodging Industry**. New York: Laventhol & Horwath, 1932-1990. Annual.

Laventhol & Horwath, a national accounting and consulting firm, disbanded in 1991 after filing for bankruptcy. The firm played a major role in analyzing various segments of the hospitality industry including lodging. This report was regarded by industry experts as the definitive source of information on the lodging industry's annual performance in this country. Data were based on responses to a mailed questionnaire. In addition to statistical data, there were articles on the lodging industry. Because this report had been compiled since the 1930s, it was an excellent source of trend data. Laventhol & Horwath also produced individual reports on segments of the U.S. lodging industry. These included: *Florida Lodging Industry*, *Texas Lodging Industry*, *California Lodging Industry*, *U.S. Resort Lodging Industry*, *U.S. Economy/Limited Service Lodging Industry*, and *All-Suite Lodging Industry*.

D-75. **Worldwide Hotel Industry**. New York: Laventhol & Horwath, 1971-1990. Annual.

This annual report calculated the median operating and financial performance of hotels around the world based on an analysis of more than 1,000 completed survey forms. All currency figures were converted to U.S. dollars. Aggregate data were presented for international hotels, but most data were regional. Detailed statistics were provided for the following regions: Africa and the Middle East; Asia and Australia; North America; Europe; and Latin America and the Caribbean. Analysts based in Laventhol & Horwath's international offices around the world offered analytical commentaries on hotel performance in individual countries and subregions, often correlating hotel performance with an increase or decrease in travel to a region.

D-76. **Yearbook of Tourism Statistics**. Madrid: World Tourism Organization, 1953- . Annual.

This annual publication summarizes important international tourism statistics in chart form and presents detailed data for approximately 150 countries. Information is published in Spanish, French, and English. Aggregate data on world tourism go back to 1950. This series began after World War II and is an important source of data on the historical development of tourism in individual countries. Data on individual countries are specific. For example, you can find the monthly occupancy rates for hotels in individual countries. In some cases, you can find a breakdown of tourism receipts—that is, how much money tourists spent on lodging, meals, transportation, recreation, shopping, etc. The source for this data is the World Tourism Organization's annual survey of official government agencies. Survey data are supplemented by statistics published in official national publications and by information obtained through additional correspondence with government agencies. This two-volume compilation represents the most complete collection of published government data on international travel and tourism.

NOTES

[1]Maxine Feifer, *Tourism in History: From Imperial Rome to the Present* (New York: Stein and Day, 1985), 8.

[2]For accounts of the history of tourism see A. J. Burkhart and S. Medlik, *Tourism: Past, Present, and Future* (London: Heinemann, 1974); Feifer, *Tourism in History*; L. J. Lickorish and A. G. Kershaw, *The Travel Trade* (London: Practical Press, 1958); Donald E. Lundberg, *The Tourist Business*, 6th ed. (New York: Van Nostrand Reinhold, 1990); Robert W. McIntosh and Charles R. Goeldner, *Tourism: Principles, Practices, Philosophies*, 6th ed. (New York: Wiley, 1989); and Louis Turner and John Ash, *The Golden Hordes: International Tourism and the Pleasure Periphery* (New York: St. Martin's, 1976).

[3]Alexander Moore, "Walt Disney World: Bounded Ritual Space and the Playful Pilgrimage Center," *Anthropological Quarterly*, 53:4 (1980): 207-18.

[4]Chuck Y. Gee, Dexter J. L. Choy, and James C. Makens, *The Travel Industry* (Westport, CT: AVI, 1984), 5.

[5]Ibid., 5.

[6]Ibid., 5-6.

[7]*Economic Review of Travel in America, 1988-89* (Washington, DC: U.S. Travel Data Center, 1988), B-1-B-2.

[8]For discussions on defining travel and tourism see Ray Bar-On, *Travel and Tourism Data: A Comprehensive Research Handbook on the World Travel Industry* (Phoenix, AZ: Oryx, 1989); Burkhart, *Tourism: Past, Present, and Future*; Robin A. Chadwick, "Concepts, Definitions and Measures Used in Travel and Tourism Research," in *Travel, Tourism, and Hospitality Research: A Handbook for Managers and Researchers*, ed. J. R. Brent Ritchie and Charles R. Goeldner (New York: Wiley, 1987): 47-61; Gee et al., *The Travel Industry*; Neil Leiper, "The Framework of Tourism: Towards a Definition of Tourism, Tourist, and the Tourist Industry," *Annals of Tourism Research*, 6:4 (1979): 390-407; Lundberg, *The Tourist Business*; and McIntosh, *Tourism: Principles, Practices, Philosophies*.

[9]John Heeley, "The Definition of Tourism in Great Britain: Does Terminological Confusion Have to Rule?" *Revue de Tourisme*, 35:2 (1980): 11-14.

[10]*Economic Review of Travel in America, 1988-89*, 13. (Reprinted by permission U.S. Travel Data Center.)

[11]Ibid., 35.

[12]Ibid., 25.

[13]Ibid., 55.

[14]Bar-On, 156.

[15]Barbara A. Weightman, "Third World Tour Landscapes," *Annals of Tourism Research*, 14:2 (1987): 227. (Reprinted with permission Pergamon Press.)

[16]For some broad discussions as well as case studies of the impacts of travel and tourism see Burkhart, *Tourism: Past, Present, and Future*; Erlet A. Cater, "Tourism in the Least Developed Countries," *Annals of Tourism Research*, 14:2 (1987): 202-26; Gee, *The Travel Industry*; Herbert G. Kariel, "Tourism and Development: Perplexity or Panacea?" *Journal of Travel Research*, 28:1 (1989): 2-6; Lundberg, *The Tourist Business*; Dean MacCannell, *The Tourist: A New Theory of the Leisure Class* (New York: Schocken, 1976); McIntosh, *Tourism: Principles, Practices, Philosophies*; J. R. Brent Ritchie, "Assessing the Impact of Hallmark Events: Conceptual and Research Issues," *Journal of Travel Research*, 23:1 (1984): 2-11; John E. Rosenow and Gerald L. Pulsipher, *Tourism: The Good, the Bad, and the Ugly* (Lincoln, NE: Century Three Press, 1979); Turner, *The Golden Hordes: International Tourism and the Pleasure Periphery*; Valene L. Smith, ed., *Hosts and Guests: The Anthropology of Tourism*, 2d ed. (Philadelphia: University of Pennsylvania Press, 1989); and Barbara A. Weightman, "Third World Tour Landscapes," *Annals of Tourism Research*, 14:2 (1987): 227-39.

[17]Cater, 208.

[18]C. R. Goeldner, "Tourism: A Vital Force for Peace," *Journal of Travel Research*, 27:3 (1989): 44. (Published by the Business Research Division, University of Colorado at Boulder and the Travel and Tourism Research Association.)

[19]Ibid., 46.

[20]Ibid., 45-46.

[21]Weightman, 231, 232, 235.

[22]Neil Leiper, "Towards a Cohesive Curriculum in Tourism: The Case for a Distinct Discipline," *Annals of Tourism Research*, 8:1 (1981): 81.

[23]Emilyn A. Sheffield and Kathleen A. Davis, "Evolution of Sport and Leisure Management: Commonalities and Crosslinkages," *Visions in Leisure and Business*, 7:1 (1988): 7.

[24]Ibid., 7.

[25]Peter E. Murphy, "Tourism Course Proposal for a Social Science Curriculum," *Annals of Tourism Research*, 8:1 (1981): 99.

[26]Graham Dann, Dennison Nash, and Philip Pearce, "Methodology in Tourism Research," *Annals of Tourism Research*, 15:1 (1988): 3.

[27]Ibid., 2.

[28]Ibid., 7.

[29]Douglas G. Pearce, "Towards a Geography of Tourism," *Annals of Tourism Research*, 6:3 (1979): 267, 268.

[30]Erik Cohen, "Rethinking the Sociology of Tourism," *Annals of Tourism Research*, 6:1 (1979): 19-20.

[31]Valene L. Smith, "Anthropology and Tourism: A Science Industry Evaluation," *Annals of Tourism Research*, 7:1 (1980): 29.

[32]Ibid., 30.

[33]For an explanation of psychographic research applied to tourism studies see Gee, *The Travel Industry*; Lundberg, *The Tourist Business*; McIntosh, *Tourism: Principles, Practices, Philosophies*; and Stanley C. Plog, "Understanding Psychographics in Tourism Research," in *Travel, Tourism, and Hospitality Research: A Handbook for Managers and Researchers*, ed. J. R. Brent Ritchie and Charles R. Goeldner (New York: Wiley, 1987): 203-13.

[34]Donald E. Lundberg, *The Tourist Business*, 5th ed. (New York: Van Nostrand Reinhold, 1985), 161.

[35]Linda K. Richter, "Tourism Politics and Political Science: A Case of Not So Benign Neglect," *Annals of Tourism Research*, 10:3 (1983): 316.

[36]Harry G. Matthews, "Editor's Page," *Annals of Tourism Research*, 10:3 (1983): 303, 304, 305. (Reprinted with permission Pergamon Press.)

[37]Anthony J. Fedler, "Are Leisure, Recreation, and Tourism Interrelated?" *Annals of Tourism Research*, 14:3 (1987): 313.

[38]Richard R. Perdue, Ann S. Coughlin, and Laura Valerius, "Tourism and Commercial Recreation: Past, Present, and Future Research," in *Proceedings of the 10th Annual Symposium on Leisure Research* (New Orleans, LA, 1987), 23.

[39]Ibid., 24.

[40]Ibid., 24.

[41]Bryan H. Farrell and Robert W. McLellan, "Tourism and Physical Environment Research," *Annals of Tourism Research*, 14:1 (1987): 9.

[42]C. R. Goeldner, *Data Sources for Tourism Research* (Boulder, CO: Business Research Division, Graduate School of Business Administration, University of Colorado, 1989), 1.

[43]Purdue et al., 24.

[44]The source of information about the Travel Economic Import Model and the activities of the U.S. Travel Data Center is a presentation delivered by Kelly Repass, Research Analyst at the U.S. Travel Data Center, at The Pennsylvania State University on April 20, 1990.

[45]Perdue et al., 24.

[46]Laurel J. Reid and Kathleen L. Andereck, "Statistical Analyses Use in Tourism Research," *Journal of Travel Research*, 28:2 (1989): 22.

[47]Ibid., 22.

[48]Ibid., 23.

[49]J. R. Brent Ritchie, "Some Critical Aspects of Measurement Theory and Practice in Travel Research," *Journal of Travel Research*, 14:1 (1975): 1-10.

[50]Ibid., 3.

[51]J. R. Brent Ritchie, "Assessing the Impact of Hallmark Events," 2-11.

[52]Charles P. Cantee and D. C. Williams, Jr., "Tourism Impacts and Rankings: Methodological Myth Economic Inquiry," *Visions in Leisure and Business*, 6:4 (1988): 11.

[53]Ibid., 12.

[54]For information about the Travel and Tourism Research Association see their brochure, *Travel and Tourism Research Association: What It Is— What It Does— Why You Should Join* (Salt Lake City, UT: TTRA, n.d.).

APPENDIX
A

DEGREE PROGRAMS

LEISURE STUDIES PROGRAMS

The following colleges and universities offer baccalaureate- and graduate-level programs or areas of specialization in leisure studies, leisure services, leisure management, recreation, and other leisure-related social science curricula. B indicates that an institution offers a baccalaureate-level program; M indicates a master's degree program; and D indicates a doctoral-level program.

American Colleges and Universities

Boston University
Leisure Studies Program
121 Bay State Road
Boston, MA 02215
(617) 353-2318
B,M,D

Central Washington University
Leisure Services Program
Ellensburg, WA 98926
(509) 963-1211
B

Christopher Newport College
Leisure Studies Program
50 Shoe Lane
Newport News, VA 23606
(804) 599-7000
B

East Carolina University
Leisure Systems Studies Program
East Fifth Street
Greenville, NC 27858-4553
(919) 757-6131
B

Florida State University
Leisure Services Program
216 BWJB
Tallahassee, FL 32303
(904) 644-6200
B,M

Green Mountain College
Leisure Management Program
16 College Street
Poultney, VT 05764
(802) 287-9313
B

Iowa State University
Leisure Services Program
Alumni Hall
Ames, IA 50011
(515) 294-5836
B

Missouri Western State College
Leisure Services Program
Newman and Duquesne Roads
Joplin, MO 64801
(417) 625-9300
B

New Mexico Highlands University
Leisure Services Program
Las Vegas, NM 87701
(505) 425-7511
B

North Dakota State University
Leisure Services Program
University Station
Fargo, ND 58105
(701) 237-7752
B

Northwestern Illinois University
Leisure Studies Program
Evanston, IL 60204
(312) 491-7271
B

Oklahoma State University
Leisure Science Program
Stillwater, OK 74078
(405) 744-5000
B

Salisbury State University
Leisure Services Program
Salisbury, MD 21801
(301) 543-6000
B

Seattle Pacific University
Leisure and Recreation Program
3307 Third Avenue West
Seattle, WA 98119
(206) 281-2051
B

University of Illinois, Urban-
    Champaign
Leisure Studies Program
506 South Wright Street
Urbana, IL 61801
(217) 333-1000
B,M,D

University of Massachusetts,
    Amherst
Leisure Studies Program
Amherst, MA 01003
(413) 545-0222
B

University of New Hampshire
Leisure Management and Tourism
    Program
Durham, NH 03824
(603) 862-1360
B

University of Oregon
Leisure Studies and Recreation
    Program
240 Oregon Hall
Eugene, OR 97403
(503) 686-3201
B,M,D

University of Tulsa
Leisure Development Program
600 South College Avenue
Tulsa, OK 74104
(918) 631-2307
B

Wartburg College
Leisure Services Program
222 Ninth Street NW
Waverly, IA 50677
(319) 325-8264
B

Canadian Colleges and Universities

Concordia University
Leisure Studies Program
1455 de Maisonneuve Boulevard West
Montreal, Quebec, Canada
    PQH3G 1M8
(514) 848-2424
B

Dalhousie University
Leisure Studies Program
Halifax, Nova Scotia, Canada
B3H 3J5
(902) 424-2211
B

Malaspina College
Leisure Studies Program
900 Fifth Street
Nanaimo, British Columbia, Canada
V9R 5S5
(604) 753-3245
B

University of Ottawa
Leisure Studies Program
550 Cumberland Street
Ottawa, Ontario, Canada K1N 6N5
(613) 564-3928
B

FITNESS AND RELATED PROGRAMS

The following colleges and universities offer baccalaureate- and graduate-level programs or areas of specialization in fitness or fitness-related programs. B indicates that an institution offers a baccalaureate-level program; M indicates a master's degree program; and D indicates a doctoral-level program.

American Colleges and Universities

Arizona State University
Department of Health and Physical Education
Tempe, AZ 85287
(602) 965-7788; (800) 252-ASUI
B,M,D

Ball State University
Department of Physiology and Health Science
Muncie, IN 47306
(317) 285-8300
B,M,D

Boston University
School of Education, Program in Human Movement
121 Bay State Road
Boston, MA 02215
(617) 353-2318
B,M,D

California State University, Chico
Department of Physical Education
1st and Normal Streets
Chico, CA 95929
(916) 895-6321
B

California State University, Los Angeles
Department of Physical Education and Recreation/Leisure Studies
515 State College Drive
Los Angeles, CA 90032
(213) 224-3361
B,M,D

Colorado State University
Department of Exercise and Sport Science
Fort Collins, CO 80523
(303) 491-1101
B,M

Frostburg State University
Department of Education, Program in Health and Physical Education
Frostburg, MD 21532
(301) 689-4201
B,M

Indiana University
School of Health, Physical Education
 and Recreation
84 East Third Street
Bloomington, IN 47401
(812) 855-0661
B,M,D

Miami University at Oxford
Department of Physical Education,
 Health, and Sports Studies
East High Street
Oxford, OH 45056
(513) 529-2531
B,M

Michigan State University
School of Health Education, Coun-
 seling Psychology, and Human
 Performance
East Lansing, MI 48824
(517) 355-8332
B,M,D

Ohio State University
School of Health, Physical Education, and Leisure Studies
1800 Cannon Drive
Columbus, OH 43210
(614) 292-3980
B,M

Pennsylvania State University
Department of Exercise and Sport
 Science
University Park, PA 16802
(814) 865-5471
B,M,D

San Diego State University
Department of Physical Education
5300 Campanile Drive
San Diego, CA 92182
(619) 594-6871
B,M

San Francisco State University
Department of Physical Education
1600 Holloway Avenue
San Francisco, CA 94132
(415) 338-2164
B,M

Teachers College, Columbia University
Department of Movement Sciences
525 West 120th Street
New York, NY 10027
(212) 678-3000
B,M,D

University of California, Berkeley
Department of Physical Education
Berkeley, CA 94720
(415) 642-6000
B,M,D

University of California, Los Angeles
Program in Kinesiology
405 Hilgard Avenue
Los Angeles, CA 90024
(213) 825-3101
B,M,D

University of Connecticut
Department of Sport and Leisure
 Studies
Storrs, CT 06268
(203) 486-3137
B,M,D

University of Florida
Department of Exercise and Sport
 Science
West University Avenue and 13th
 Street
Gainsville, FL 32611
(904) 392-3261
B,M,D

University of Houston
Department of Health, Physical
 Education and Recreation
4800 Calhoun Boulevard
Houston, TX 77004
(713) 749-1011
B,M,D

University of Illinois, Urbana-
 Champaign
Department of Kinesiology
506 South Wright Street
Urbana, IL 61801
(217) 333-1000
B,M,D

University of Iowa
Department of Physical Education
and Sports Studies
Iowa City, IA 52242
(319) 335-3847
B,M,D

University of Massachusetts,
Amherst
School of Physical Education, Exercise Science Program
Amherst, MA 01003
(413) 545-0222
B,M,D

University of Michigan
School of Education
Division of Physical Education
Ann Arbor, MI 48109
(313) 764-7433
B,M,D

University of Montana
Department of Health and Physical
Education
Missoula, MT 59801
(406) 243-6266
B,M

University of North Carolina,
Greensboro
Department of Physical Education
1000 Spring Garden Street
Greensboro, NC 27412
(919) 334-5000
B,M,D

University of Texas, Austin
Department of Kinesiology and
Health Education
Austin, TX 78713
(512) 471-3434
B,M,D

University of Wisconsin, La Crosse
Department of Physical Education
1725 State Street
La Crosse, WI 54601
(608) 785-8000
B

University of Wisconsin, Milwaukee
Program in Human Kinetics
P.O. Box 413
Milwaukee, WI 53201
(414) 229-3800
B,M

University of Wisconsin, Stevens
Point
School of Health, Physical Education, Recreation and Athletics
2100 Main Street
Stevens Point, WI 54481
(715) 346-2441
B

Canadian Colleges and Universities

Laval University/Université Laval
Cité Universitaire
Ste-Foy, Quebec, Canada
PQG1K 7P4
(418) 656-2131
B,M,D

McMaster University
1280 Main Street West
Hamilton, Ontario, Canada L8S 4L8
(416) 525-9140
B

University of Alberta
Department of Physical Education
Edmonton, Alberta, Canada
T5G 2E1
(403) 432-3111
B,M,D

University of Toronto
Toronto, Ontario, Canada M5S 1A1
(416) 978-2011
B,M,D

University of Windsor
Faculty of Human Kinetics
401 Sunset Avenue
Windsor, Ontario, Canada N9B 3P4
(519) 253-4232
B

SPORT AND RELATED PROGRAMS

The following colleges and universities offer baccalaureate- and graduate-level programs or areas of specialization in sports and sports-related programs. B indicates that an institution offers a baccalaureate-level program; M indicates a master's degree program; and D indicates a doctoral-level program. This list is by no means comprehensive.

American Colleges and Universities

Arizona State University
Department of Exercise Science
Tempe, AZ 85287-0112
(602) 965-7788
B,M,D

Arkansas State University
Department of Sports Science
P.O. Box 1630
State University, AK 72467
(501) 972-2031
B

Atlantic Christian College
Department of Sports Science
A.C.C. Station Wilson, NC 27893
(800) 345-4973
B

Brooklyn College
The City University of New York
Department of Sports Science
Bedford and H Avenue
Brooklyn, NY 11210
(718) 780-5485
M

California State University, Fullerton
Department of Sports Science
P-180, Gym
Fullerton, CA 92634
(714) 773-2676
B,M

Campbell University
Department of Sports and Fitness
Buies Creek, NC 27506
(919) 893-4111
B

Central Michigan University
Department of Physical Education
  and Sports
Rose Center
Mt. Pleasant, MI 48859
(517) 774-6659
B,M

Chapman College
Department of Sports Medicine
333 North Glassell Street
Orange, CA 92666
(714) 997-6711
M

Columbus College
Department of Physical Education/
  Leisure Management
Columbus, GA 31993-2399
(404) 568-2046
B,M

Eastern Kentucky University
EKU College of HPER&A
Weaver Building
202 Richmond, KY 40475
(606) 622-1887
B,M

Georgia Southern College
Department of Sport Science and
  Physical Education
LB 8076
Statesboro, GA 30460
(912) 681-5266
M

Georgia State University
Department of HPRD
University Plaza
Atlanta, GA 30303
(404) 651-2536
B,M

Grambling State University
Department of Sports Science
Campus Box 871
Grambling, LA 71245
(318) 274-2712
B,M

Guilford College
Department of Sports Science
5800 West Friendly Avenue
Greensboro, NC 27410
(919) 292-5511
B

Keene State College
Department of Sports Science/
    Department of Physical
    Education
229 Main Street
Keene, NH 03431
(603) 352-1909, ext. 333
B

Kent State University
Department of Sport Science
School of Health, Physical Educa-
    tion, and Recreation
264 Memorial Annex
Kent, OH 44242
(216) 672-2990
B,M,D

Loras College
Department of Sport Science
1450 Alta Vista Drive
Dubuque, IA 52001
(319) 558-7196
B,M

Marshall University
Division of Health, Physical Educa-
    tion, and Recreation
College of Education
Huntington, WV 25701
(304) 696-6490
B

Michigan State University
Department of Health Education/
    Human Performance
232 Jenison
East Lansing, MI 48824
(517) 355-1642
B,M,D

Montana State University
Department of Sports Science
Room 225 Romney Gym
Bozeman, MT 59717
(406) 994-4001
B,M

Northeastern University
Department of Sports Science
360 Huntington Avenue
3 Dockser Hall
Boston, MA 02115
(617) 437-3166
B,M

Ohio State University
Sport Management Program
School of Health, Physical Educa-
    tion, and Recreation
249 Larkins Hall
337 West 17th Avenue
Columbus, OH 43210-1284
(614) 292-7701
B,M,D

Ohio University
Department of Sports Science
Grover Center
Athens, OH 45701
(614) 593-4666
B,M

Oregon State University
Department of Sports Science
Corvallis, OR 97331
(503) 754-4411
B

Penn State University
Department of Exercise and Sport
    Science
105 White Building
University Park, PA 16802
(814) 863-1289
B,M,D

Pfeiffer College
Department of Sports Science
Misenheimer, NC 28109
(704) 463-7343
B

Robert Morris College
Department of Sports Management
Narrows Run Road
Coraopolis, PA 15108-1189
(412) 262-8302
B,M

Saint Olaf College
Department of Exercise Science
Northfield, MN 55057
(507) 663-2222
B

Salem State College
Department of Sports Science
352 Lafayette Street
Salem, MA 01970
(508) 254-2610
B

Slippery Rock University of
    Pennsylvania
Department of Physical Education/
    HMS
Maltby Center
Slippery Rock, PA 16057
(412) 794-7203
B,M

Southern Illinois University,
    Carbondale
Department of Physical Education/
    HMS
Athletics-Davies 160
Carbondale, IL 62901
B,M,D

Springfield College
Department of Sport Science
263 Alden Street
Springfield, MA 01109
(413) 788-3275
B,M

State University of New York,
    Buffalo
Department of Sport and Exercise
    Studies
3435 Main Street
Buffalo, NY 14214
(716) 831-2000
B,M,D

United States Sports Academy
One Academy Drive
Dapheny, AL 36426
(205) 626-3303; Fax (205) 626-3874
M

University of Arizona
Department of Exercise Science
Tucson, AZ 85721
(602) 621-3237
M

University of Connecticut
Department of Sport/Leisure &
    Exercise Sciences
2111 Hillside Road U-110
Storrs, CT 06269-3100
(203) 486-3623
B,M,D

University of Florida
Department of Exercise and Sports
    Science
West University Avenue & 13th Street
303 Florida Gym
Gainesville, FL 32611
(904) 392-0584
B,M,D

University of Illinois, Urbana-
 Champaign
Department of Physical Education/
 HMS
170 IMPE Building
201 Peabody Drive
Champaign, IL 61820
(217) 333-9780
B,M,D

University of Indiana
Department of Physical Education
HPER Building
Suite 112 (Undergraduate)
Suite 179 (Master's)
Bloomington, IN 47405
(821) 335-1230
B,M

University of Maryland
Department of Physical Education
College Park, MD 20742
(301) 454-4916
B,M

University of Massachusetts,
 Amherst
Department of Sports Science
Curry Hickes Building
Room #1
Amherst, MA 01002
(413) 545-2336
B,M,D

University of Mississippi
Department of Health, Physical Edu-
 cation, and Recreation
Turner Complex
University, MS 38677
(601) 232-5521
B,M

University of Richmond
Department of Sports Science
Robins Center
Richmond, VA 23173
(804) 289-8350
M

University of South Carolina
College of Applied Professional
 Sciences
Sports Administration Department
Carolina Coliseum, Room 2012
Columbia, SC 29208
(803) 777-4690
B

University of Southern California
Department of Sports Science
University Park
Los Angeles, CA 90089-0911
(213) 743-6741
B

University of Texas
Kinesiology and Health Education
 Department
Bellmont 222
Austin, TX 78712
(512) 471-3434
M

West Virginia University
Department of Sports Science
P.O. Box 6116
265 Coliseum
Morgantown, WV 26506-6116
(304) 293-3295
B,M

TRAVEL AND TOURISM PROGRAMS

The following colleges and universities offer baccalaureate- and graduate-level programs or areas of specialization in travel and tourism management. Travel and tourism courses are also offered in general hospitality programs and in geography, recreation and parks, and other social science curricula. B indicates that an institution offers a baccalaureate-level program; M indicates a master's degree program; and D indicates a doctoral-level program.

Alaska Pacific University
Travel and Hospitality Management
4101 University Drive
Anchorage, AK 99508
(907) 561-1266
B

Belmont College
Tourism Management
1900 Belmont Boulevard
Nashville, TN 37212-3757
(615) 383-7001
B

Bethune-Cookman College
Hospitality Management Program
Division of Business
640 Second Avenue
Daytona Beach, FL 32015
(904) 255-1401
B

Black Hills State University
Travel Industry Management
1200 University Avenue
Box 9502
Spearfish, SD 57783
(605) 692-6011
B

Boston University
School of Hotel and Food Adminis-
    tration
808 Commonwealth Avenue
Boston, MA 02215
(617) 353-3261
B

Brigham Young University, Hawaii
Hotel, Restaurant, and Travel
    Management
Laie, HI 96762
(808) 293-3588
B

College of Boca Raton
Hotel, Restaurant and Tourism
    Management
509 Wixted Hall
3601 North Military Trail
Boca Raton, FL 33431
(407) 994-0770
B

Columbia College
Travel Administration
10th and Rogers
Columbia, MO 65216
(800) 231-2391
B

Concord College
Travel Industry Management
Athens, WV 24712
(304) 384-3115, ext. 5263
B

Davis and Elkins College
Travel and Tourism
100 Sycamore Street
Elkins, WV 26241
(304) 636-1900
B

East Stroudsburg University
Hospitality Management
East Stroudsburg, PA 18301
(717) 424-3511
B

Fairleigh Dickinson University
School of Hotel, Restaurant and
    Tourism Management
180 Fairview Avenue
Rutherford, NJ 07070
(201) 460-5362
B

George Washington University
Tourism Administration Program
817 23rd Street, NW
Washington, DC 20052
(202) 994-6280
B,M,D

Georgia Southern College
Hospitality Administration, Hotel
    and Tourism Management
Statesboro, GA 30460-8034
(912) 681-5345
B

Golden Gate University
Hotel, Restaurant, Institutional and
    Tourism Program
536 Mission Street
San Francisco, CA 94105
(415) 442-7215
B

Hawaii Pacific College
Travel Industry Management
1188 Fort Street, Fourth Floor
Honolulu, HI 98813
(808) 544-0228
B

Houston-Tillotson College
Department of Business Administra-
    tion and Economics
1820 East 8th Street
Austin, TX 78702
(512) 476-7421
B

Johnson & Wales University
Hospitality Program
Abbott Park Place
Providence, RI 02903
(401) 456-1475
B

Kearney State College
Tourism and Travel
Business College
Kearney, NE 68849-0605
(308) 234-8515
B

Mansfield University of Pennsylvania
Travel/Tourism
Beecher House
Mansfield, PA 16933
(717) 662-4000
B

Michigan State University
School of Hotel, Restaurant and
    Institutional Management
424 Eppley Center
East Lansing, MI 48824-1121
(517) 355-5080
B

Morris Brown College
Hotel, Restaurant and Tourism
    Management
643 Martin Luther King, Jr.,
    Drive, NW
Atlanta, GA 30314
(404) 525-7831
B

National College
Travel and Tourism Management
321 Kansas City Street
Box 1780
Rapid City, SD 57709
(605) 394-4800
B

New School for Social Research,
    Eugene Lange College
Travel and Tourism Management
65 West 11th Street
New York, NY 10111
(212) 741-5950
M

Niagara University
Institute of Travel, Hotel and Restau-
    rant Administration
Niagara, NY 14109
(716) 285-1212, ext. 375
B

Northeastern State University
Tourism Management
Tahlequah, OK 74464
(918) 456-5511
B

Northern Arizona University
School of Hotel and Restaurant
    Management
Flagstaff, AZ 86011
(602) 523-2845
B

Oregon State University
Hotel, Restaurant and Tourism
    Management Program
Corvallis, OR 97331-2603
(503) 754-3693
B

Parks College of St. Louis University
Travel and Tourism
Cahokia, IL 62206
(618) 337-7500, ext. 210
B

Purdue University
Restaurant, Hotel and Institutional
    Management
105 Stone Hall
West Lafayette, IN 47907
(317) 494-4600
B,M

Rochester Institute of Technology
School of Food, Hotel and Tourism
    Management
Rochester, NY 14623
(716) 475-5576
B,M

Saint Thomas University
Tourism and Hospitality Manage-
    ment
College of Business
16400 Northwest 32nd Avenue
Miami, FL 33054
(305) 628-6627
B

Sierra Nevada College, Lake Tahoe
P.O. Box 4269
800 College Drive
Incline Village, NV 89450-4269
(702) 831-1314
B

Texas A & M University
Tourism Management
Department of Recreation and Parks
College Station, TX 77843-2261
(409) 845-7324
B,M,D

United States International
    University
Hospitality Management
10455 Pomerado Road
San Diego, CA 92131
(619) 271-4300
B

University of Alaska, Fairbanks
Travel Industry Management
    Program
School of Management
Fairbanks, AK 99775-1070
(907) 474-6528
B,M

University of Central Florida
Hospitality Management
Orlando, FL 32816
(407) 275-2188
B

University of Hawaii, Manoa
School of Travel Industry Manage-
    ment
2560 Campus Road
Honolulu, HI 96822
(808) 948-8111
B,M

University of Houston
Conrad Hilton College
4800 Calhoun Drive
Houston, TX 77004
(713) 749-1451
B,M

University of Massachusetts,
    Amherst
Department of Hotel, Restaurant
    and Travel Administration
Flint Lab
Amherst, MA 01003
(413) 545-2535
B,M

University of Nevada, Las Vegas
College of Hotel Administration
4505 Maryland Parkway
Las Vegas, NV 89154
(702) 739-3230
B,M

The University of New Haven
Hotel, Restaurant and Tourism
    Administration
300 Orange Avenue
West Haven, CT 06516
(203) 932-7000
B,M

The University of New Mexico
Travel & Tourism Management
    Program
Anderson School of Management
University of New Mexico
Albuquerque, NM 87131
(505) 277-3403
B

University of New Orleans
School of Hotel, Restaurant and
    Tourism Management
College of Business Administration
New Orleans, LA 70148
(504) 286-6385
B

University of South Carolina
Hotel, Restaurant and Tourism
    Administration
Columbia, SC 29208
(803) 777-6665
B

University of Southern Mississippi
Hotel and Restaurant Administration
Southern Station
Box 5035
Hattiesburg, MS 39406-5035
(601) 266-4906
B,M

University of Tennessee
Department of Tourism, Food and
    Lodging Administration
College of Human Ecology
220 CHE
Knoxville, TN 37996
(615) 974-1000
B

University of Wisconsin, Stout
Hotel and Restaurant Management
220 Home Economics
Menomonie, WI 54571
(715) 232-1405
B,M

Villa Maria College
Tourism and Recreational Manage-
    ment
2551 West Lake Road
Erie, PA 16505-4494
(814) 838-5332
B

Virginia Polytechnic Institute and
    State University
Hotel, Restaurant and Institutional
    Management
Hillcrest Hall
Blacksburg, VA 24061-0429
(703) 231-5515
B,M,D

Webber College
Business Administration Department
Route 27-A
Babson Park, FL 33827
(813) 638-1431
B

Western Michigan University
Travel and Tourism
Department of Geography
Kalamazoo, MI 49008
(616) 387-3410
B

IMPORTANT PUBLISHERS

LEISURE STUDIES

CAB International
Wallingford, Oxon, UK 10 8DE
Telex 847964; Tel. Wallingford
  (0491) 32111
Fax 0491 33508

Charles C. Thomas, Publisher
2600 South First Street
Springfield, IL 62794-9265
(217) 789-8980

John Wiley and Sons, Inc.
605 Third Avenue
New York, NY 10158
(212) 850-6000

Open University Press
1900 Front Road, Suite 101
Bristol, PA 19007
(215) 985-5800; (800) 821-8312

Routledge and Kegan Paul, Ltd.
London, UK EC4
Telex 263398; Tel. 01-583 9855
Fax 01 583-0701

University Press of America, Inc.
4720 Boston Way
Lanham, MD 20706
(301) 459-3366

Unwin Hyman, Ltd. (formerly Allen
  & Unwin)
15-17 Broadwich Street
London, UK W1V 1FP
Telex 23732; Tel. 01-439 3126
Fax 01734-3884

Venture Publishing, Inc.
1640 Oxford Circle
State College, PA 16801
(814) 234-4561

W. B. Saunders Company
The Curtis Center
Independence Square West
Philadelphia, PA 19106
(215) 238-7800

William C. Brown Group
2460 Kerper Boulevard
Dubuque, IA 52001
(319) 588-1451; (800) 338-5578

FITNESS AND RELATED SUBJECTS

Aerobics and Fitness Association of
  America
15250 Ventura Boulevard, Suite 310
Sherman Oaks, CA 91403
(818) 905-0040

Videos, magazines, texts, and work-
books.

American Alliance for Health, Physical Education, Recreation, and Dance (AAHPERD)
P.O. Box 704
Waldorf, MD 20604
(703) 476-3481, 3400

Periodicals, books, texts, resource kits, audiovisuals, software, and personalized sportswear.

American College of Sports Medicine (ACSM)
401 West Michigan Street
P.O. Box 1440
Indianapolis, IN 46206
(317) 637-9200; Fax (317) 634-7817

Newsmagazine, career newsletter, journal, reference guides, and position papers.

American Demographics Press
P.O. Box 68
Ithaca, NY 14851
(800) 828-1133

Consumer marketing information: books, magazines, newsletters, and catalog for marketing executives.

American Health Consultants
60 Peachtree Park Drive
Atlanta, GA
(800) 554-1032; In Georgia:
    (404) 351-4523

Newsletters and reports for health care professionals.

Benchmark Press, Inc.
701 Congressional Boulevard
Suite 340
Carmel, IN 46032
(312) 573-6420; Fax (317) 573-6424

Books, texts, journals, videos, software, and instructional program kits.

Human Kinetics Publishers, Inc.
Box 5076
Champaign, IL 61825-5076
(800) 747-4457; Fax (217) 351-2674

Books, texts, journals, videotapes, instructor's guides, test manuals, study guides, and software.

Institute for Aerobics Research
12330 Preston Road
Dallas, TX 75230
(214) 701-8001

Newsletters, books, research studies, handbooks, software, and texts/ assessments.

Lea & Febiger
Chester Field Parkway
Malvern, PA 19355
(215) 251-2230

Medical and clinical texts.

Leisure Press
(Division of Human Kinetics
    Publishers)
Box 5076
Champaign, IL 61825-5076
(800) 747-4457 or (217) 351-5076

Books and videos.

National Center for Health Statistics
Department of Health and Human
    Services
Center Building, Room 1-57
3700 East-West Highway
Hyattsville, MD 20782
(301) 436-7135

Vital statistics on such subjects as health care delivery, health resources utilization, families and dental health.

ODPHP National Health Information Center
P.O. Box 1133
Washington, DC 20013-1133
(800) 336-4797; In Maryland:
    (301) 565-4167

Information on government programs and policies related to community health promotion, school health, worksite health, nutrition, professional education, education materials and other issues.

Oryx Press
2214 North Central at Encanto
Phoenix, AZ 85004
(800) 457-ORYX; Fax (602) 253-2741

Books, reference tools, and hand-books.

President's Council on Physical Fitness and Sports
450 Fifth Street, NW
Suite 7103
Washington, DC 20001
(202) 272-3430

Monographs, newsletter, and bibliog-raphies.

Rodale Press, Inc.
33 East Minor Street
Emmaus, PA 18098
(800) 527-8200 or (215) 967-5171

Books, magazines, and newsletters.

Sport Information Resource Center
(SIRC)
1600 Promenade James Naismith
Drive
Gloucester, Ontario, Canada
K1B 5N4
(613) 748-5658; Fax (613) 748-5701

Thesaurus, bibliographies, and online database.

Washington Business Group on
Health
Prevention Leadership Forum
777 North Capitol Street, NE
Suite 800
Washington, DC 20002
(202) 408-9320; Fax (202) 408-9332

"Worksite Wellness" reports.

SPORT AND RELATED SUBJECTS

Addison-Wesley
1 Jacob Way
Reading, MA 01867
(800) 447-2226

The Athletic Institute
200 North Castlewood Drive
North Palm Beach, FL 33408
(407) 842-3600

Cambridge Physical Education and
Health
P.O. Box 2153, Department PE4
Charleston, WV 25328-2153
(800) 468-4227

Human Kinetics Publishers,
Incorporated
Box 5076
Champaign, IL 61825-5076
(800) 747-4457; Fax (217) 351-2674

Lea & Febriger
600 South Washington Square
Philadelphia, PA 19106-4158
(800) 444-1785

Leisure Press (Division of Human
Kinetics Books)
Box 5076
Champaign, IL 61825-5076
(800) 747-4457

MacGregor Sports Education Library
150 South Calhoun Road
Waukesha, WI 53186
(414) 786-0366

Sports on Video
1427 Third Street Promenade
Suite 105
Santa Monica, CA 90401
(213) 393-3358; Fax (213) 394-3136

TRAVEL
AND TOURISM

American Express Publishing
Corporation
1120 Avenue of the Americas
New York, NY 10036
(212) 382-5600

Appalachian Associates
615 Pasteur Avenue
Bowling Green, OH 43402

Association Internationale d'Experts
Scientifiques du Tourisme
Varnbüelstrasse 19
CH-9000
St. Gallen, Switzerland
071 23 55 11

Brigham Young University, Hawaii
Campus
Business Division
Box 1773
Laie, HI 96762
(808) 293-3211

Butterworth Scientific, Ltd.
P.O. Box 63
Westbury House, Bury Street
Guildford, Surrey, England
GU2 5BH
0483-300966; Fax 0483-301563

C.A.B. International
Wallingford, Oxon, England
OX10 8DE
0491-32111; Fax 0491-33508

Centre des Hautes Études
Touristiques
Université d'Aix-Marseille III
Fondation Vasarely
1 Av. Marcel Pagnol
13090 Aix-en-Provence, France
42-20-09-73

The Consortium of Hospitality
Research Information Services
c/o Information Center Publications
American Hotel & Motel Association
1201 New York Avenue
Washington, DC 20005-3917
(202) 289-3196

Cornell University
School of Hotel Administration
Statler Hall
Ithaca, NY 14853
(607) 255-5093

Council on Hotel, Restaurant and
Institutional Education
1200 17th Street, NW, 7th Floor
Washington, DC 20036-3097
(202) 331-5990; Fax (202) 331-2429

Delmar Publishers
2 Computer Drive West
Albany, NY 12205
(518) 459-1150

The Economist Publications, Ltd.
40 Duke Street
London, England WIM 5DG
01-493-6711

Euromonitor Publications, Ltd.
87-88 Turnmill Street
London, England ECIM 5QU
01-251-8024

Fairchild Books
825 Seventh Avenue
New York, NY 10019
(212) 575-9000; Fax (212) 887-1865

H. W. Wilson Co.
950 University Avenue
Bronx, NY 10452
(212) 588-8400

Information Access Company
362 Lakeside Drive
Foster City, CA 94404
(800) 227-8431

John Wiley & Sons, Inc.
605 Third Avenue
New York, NY 10158-0012
(212) 850-6418

Laventhol & Horwath
1845 Walnut Street
Philadelphia, PA 19103
(215) 299-1600

Murdoch Magazines
500 Plaza Drive
Secaucus, NJ 07096
(201) 902-2000

National Recreation and Park
Association
3101 Park Center Drive
Alexandria, VA 22302
(703) 820-4940; Fax (703) 671-4628

OECD Publications and Information
Center
1750 Pennsylvania Avenue, NW
Suite 1207
Washington, DC 20006
(202) 647-2469

Oryx Press
2214 North Central Avenue
Phoenix, AZ 85004-1483
(602) 254-6156

Pannell Kerr Forster
262 North Belt East
Houston, TX 77060
(713) 999-5134

Pergamon Press, Inc.
Journals Division
Maxwell House
Fairview Park
Elmsford, NY 10523
(914) 592-7700

Predicasts
11001 Cedar Avenue
Cleveland, OH 44106
(800) 321-6388

Prentice-Hall
Route 9W
Englewood Cliffs, NJ 07632
(201) 592-2000

Public Affairs Information Service,
Inc.
521 West 43rd Street, 5th Floor
New York, NY 10036
(212) 736-6629; Fax (212) 643-2848

Purdue University
The Restaurant, Hotel, and Institutional Management Institute
West Lafayette, IN 47907
(317) 494-2749

Schocken
201 East 50th Street
New York, NY 10022
(212) 572-2588

St. Martin's Press
175 Fifth Avenue
New York, NY 10010
(212) 674-5151

Taylor & Francis
79 Madison Avenue
New York, NY 10016
(212) 725-1999; Fax (212) 213-8368

Travel and Tourism Research
Association
P.O. Box 8066, Foothill Station
Salt Lake City, UT 84108
(801) 581-3351

United States Travel Data Center
1133 21st Street, NW
Two Lafayette Center
Washington, DC 20036
(202) 293-1040

University of Colorado
Business Research Division
Campus Box 420
Boulder, CO 80309
(303) 492-8227

University of Pennsylvania Press
418 Service Drive
Blockley Hall, 13th Floor
Philadelphia, PA 19104-6097
(215) 898-6261

University of Surrey
Library
Guildford, Surrey, England
    GU2 5XH
0483-571281, ext. 3311

Van Nostrand Reinhold
115 Fifth Avenue
New York, NY 10003
(212) 254-3232

Wakeman/Walworth, Inc.
300 North Washington Street
Suite 204
Alexandria, VA 22314
(703) 549-8606

World Tourism Organization
Captain Haya 42
28020 Madrid, Spain
5710628; Fax 5713733

LEISURE-RELATED ASSOCIATIONS

LEISURE STUDIES

American Association for Leisure and Recreation (AALR)
1900 Association Drive
Reston, VA 22091
(703) 476-3472

Commission on Education of the World Leisure and Recreation Association (CEWLRA)
P.O. Box 309
Sharbot Lake, Ontario, Canada KQH 2PO
(613) 279-3172

Commission on Research of the World Leisure and Recreation Association (CRWLRA)
1200 Mayfair Road
Champaign, IL 61821
(217) 352-3801

European Centre for Leisure and Education (ECLW)
Jilska 1
CS-11000 Prague, Czechoslovakia
2-262078

European Leisure and Recreation Association
Seefeldstrasse #8 Postfach CH-8022
Zurich, Switzerland 1 2517244

Institute of Leisure and Amnesty Management (ILAM)
Lower Basildon
Berkshire, England RG8 9NE

International Association for Social Tourism and Worker's Leisure (IASTWL)
Na Parici 15
CS110 00 Prague 1, Czechoslovakia
2-2315762

National Recreation and Parks Association (NRPA)
3101 Park Center Drive, 12th Floor
Alexandria, VA 22302
(703) 820-4940

World Leisure and Recreation Association (WLRA)
P.O. Box 309
Sharbot Lake, Ontario, Canada KDH 2PO
(613) 279-3172

FITNESS AND RELATED DISCIPLINES

Aerobics & Fitness Association of America (AFAA)
15250 Ventura Boulevard, Suite 310
Sherman Oaks, CA 91403
(818) 905-0040; (800) 445-5950

American Alliance for Health, Physical Education, Recreation and Dance (AAHPERD)
1900 Association Drive
Reston, VA 22091
(703) 476-3400

American Association for World Health (AAWH)
2001 S Street NW
Suite 530
Washington, DC 20009
(202) 265-0286

American College of Sports Medicine (ACSM)
P.O. Box 1440
Indianapolis, IN 46206
(317) 637-9200; Fax (317) 634-7817

American Fitness Association (AFA)
6700 East Pacific Coast Highway
Suite 299
Long Beach, CA 90803
(213) 596-6036

American Running and Fitness Association (AR&FA)
9310 Old Georgetown Road
Bethesda, MD 20814
(301) 897-0197

Association for Fitness in Business (AFB)
310 North Alabama Street
Suite A100
Indianapolis, IN 46204
(317) 636-6621

Association for Health and Fitness in Business
965 Hope Street
Stamford, CT 06902
(203) 359-2188

Association of Physical Fitness Centers (APFC)
600 Jefferson Street
Suite 202
Rockville, MD 20852
(301) 424-7744

The Conference Board
845 Third Avenue
New York, NY 10003
(212) 732-0882

The Institute for Aerobics Research (IAR)
12330 Preston Road
Dallas, TX 75230
(214) 701-8001

International Dance-Exercise Association (IDEA)
6190 Cornerstone Court East
Suite 204
San Diego, CA 92121
(619) 535-8979

Jazzercise
2808 Roosevelt Street
Carlsbad, CA 92008
(619) 434-2101

La Crosse Exercise and Health Program and the Wisconsin Heart Institute
221 Mitchell Hall
University of Wisconsin, La Crosse
La Crosse, WI 54601
(608) 785-8686

National Association Governor's Council on Physical Fitness and Sports (NAGCPFS)
Pan American Plaza
201 South Capitol Avenue
Suite 440
Indianapolis, IN 46225
(317) 237-5630

National Employee Services and Recreation Association (NESRA)
2400 South Downing Avenue
Westchester, IL 60153
(312) 562-8130

National Fitness Foundation (NFF)
2250 East Imperial Highway
Suite 412
El Segundo, CA 90245
(213) 640-0145

National Handicapped Sports and Recreation Association (NHSRA)

[Mailing Address]
1145 19th Street NW
Suite 717
Washington, DC 20036
(202) 783-1441

[Executive Office]
4405 East-West Highway
Suite 603
Bethesda, MD 20814
(301) 652-7505

National Health Information Clearinghouse
P.O. Box 1133
Washington, DC 20013
(301) 565-4167

National Institute for Fitness and Sport
901 West New York
Indianapolis, IN 46223
(317) 274-3432

National Strength and Conditioning Association (NSCA)
300 Old City Hall Landmark
916 O Street
P.O. Box 81410
Lincoln, NE 68501
(402) 472-3000

National Wellness Association (NWA)
South Hall
Stevens Point, WI 54481
(715) 346-2172

President's Council on Physical Fitness and Sports (PCPFS)
450 5th Street, NW
Suite 7103
Washington, DC 20001
(202) 272-3421

Washington Business Group on Health
229 Pennsylvania Avenue, SE
Washington, DC 20003
(202) 408-9320; Fax (202) 408-9332

YMCA of the USA
101 North Wacker Drive
Chicago, IL 60606
(312) 977-0031

SPORT AND RELATED DISCIPLINES

Business/Marketing

College Sports Information Directors of America
Box 114
Texas A & I University
Kingsville, TX 78363
(512) 595-3908

National Association of Concession-aires
35 East Wacker Drive
Suite 1545
Chicago, IL 60601
(312) 236-3858

Coaching

Black Coaches Association
c/o Rudy Washington, Exec. Director
P.O. Box 5371
Coralville, IA 52241
(319) 337-9595

Coaching Association of Canada
1600 James Naismith Drive
Gloucester, Ontario, Canada
K1B 5N4
(613) 748-5624; Fax (613) 758-5707

National High School Athletic
Coaches Association
Box 941329
Maitland, FL 32794-1329
(407) 628-8555

Disabled

Canadian Federation of Sports Organizations for the Disabled
1600 James Naismith Drive
Gloucester, Ontario, Canada
K1B 5N4
(613) 748-5630; Fax (613) 748-5706

National Handicapped Sports and
Recreation Association
1145 19th Street, NW
Suite 717
Washington, DC 20036
(301) 652-7505

National Wheelchair Athletic
Association
3595 East Fountain Boulevard
Suite L-10
Colorado Springs, CO 80910
(719) 574-1150

Institutional, Academic Associations

National Christian College Athletic
Association (NCCAA)
P.O. Box 1312
Marion, IN 46952
(317) 674-8401

National Collegiate Athletic Association (NCAA)
6201 College Boulevard
Overland Park, KS 66211
(913) 339-1906

National Interscholastic Athletic
Administrators Association
(NIAAA)
P.O. Box 20626
11724 Plaza Circle
Kansas City, MO 64195
(816) 464-5400

National Intramural-Recreation
Sport Association
850 SW 15th Street
Corvallis, OR 97333
(503) 754-2088

National Junior College Athletic
Association
P.O. Box 7305
Colorado Springs, CO 80933-7305
(719) 590-9788

United States Athletes Association
(USAA)
3735 Lakeland Avenue N
Suite 230
Minneapolis, MN 55422
(612) 533-5844

International

Academy of Sport Psychology
International
6079 Northgate Road
Columbus, OH 43229
(614) 846-2275

American Council on International
Sports
817 23rd Street NW
Washington, DC 20052
(202) 994-7246

General Association of International
Sports Federations Association
Générale des Federations Internationales de Sports
(GAISF/AGFIS)
Villa Henri
7, Boulevard de Suisse
MC-98000 Monte Carlo, Monaco
93 507413; Fax 33 93 25 28 73;
Telex AGFIMO 479459 MC

International Amateur Athletic
Federation
3 Hans Crescent
Knightsbridge, London, England
SW1X 0LN
71 5818771; Fax 1 5897373

International Association for Non-
Violent Sport
Stude Louis II
2, Avenue Prince Hereditaire Albert
MC-98000
Monte Carlo, Monaco
93 303649

International Association for Sports
Information
c/o Clearinghouse
Ravenstein Galery 4-27
B-1000 Brussels, Belgium
2 5135164; Fax 2 5144910

International Collegiate Sports
Foundation
P.O. Box 866
Plano, TX 75074
(214) 424-8227

International Council for Health,
Physical Education and Recreation (ICHPER)
1900 Association Drive
Reston, VA 22091
(703) 476-3400

International Society of Sports
Psychology (ISSP)
c/o Prof. Glyn Roberts
Department of Kinesiology
906 Goodwin Avenue
University of Illinois, Urbana-
Champaign
Urbana, IL 61801
(217) 244-3982

International Sports Management,
Inc.
18 West Colony Place
Suite 140
Durham, NC 27705
(919) 493-8185

Special Olympics International
1350 New York Avenue NW
Suite 500
Washington, DC 20005
(202) 628-3630; Fax (202) 737-1937

Sport for All Clearing House
44, Boulevard Leopold II
B-1080 Brussels, Belgium
2 4132891; Fax 2 4132890

Law

Sports Lawyers Association
c/o REI Management Group
2017 Lathrop Avenue
Racine, WI 53405
(414) 632-4040

Leisure and Recreation

American Association for Leisure
and Recreation
1900 Association Drive
Reston, VA 22091
(703) 476-3472

Canadian Intramural Recreation
Association
1600 James Naismith Drive
Gloucester, Ontario, Canada
K1B 5N4
(613) 748-5639; Fax (613) 748-5706

Management

College Athletic Business Managers
Association
c/o Janet Lacasse
19009-398 Laurel Park Road
Rancho Dominguez, CA 90220
(213) 637-0560

National Association of Collegiate
Directors of Athletics
P.O. Box 1648
Cleveland, OH 44116
(216) 892-4000

National Association of Intercollegiate Athletics (NAIA)
1221 Baltimore Avenue
Kansas City, MO 64105
(816) 842-5050; Fax (816) 421-4471

North American Society for Sport
Management
c/o Dr. David Matthews, President
170 IMPE 201
Peabody Drive
University of Illinois, Urbana-
Champaign
Urbana, IL 61820
(217) 333-4780

Media

American Sportscasters Association,
Inc.
5 Beekman Street
Suite 814
New York, NY 10038
(212) 227-8080

National Sportscaster and Sports
Writers Association
Box 559
Salisbury, NC 28144
(704) 633-4275

Miscellaneous

Amateur Athletic Union of the
United States (AAU)
AAU House
3400 West 86th Street
P.O. Box 68207
Indianapolis, IN 46268-0207
(317) 872-2900; Fax (317) 875-0548

Center for Sports Sponsorship
P.O. Box 280
Plainsboro, NJ 08536
(609) 924-0319

International Association of Sports
Museum and Hall of Fame
101 West Sutton Place
Wilmington, DE 19810
(202) 475-7068

National Congress of State Games
P.O. Box 2318
Billings, MT 59103
(406) 245-8106

U.S. National Senior Sport Organization
14323 South Outer 40 Road
Suite N-300
Chesterfield, MO 63017
(314) 878-4900

Officiating

National Association of Sports
Officials
2017 Lathrop Avenue
Racine, WI 53405
(414) 632-5448

Olympics

United States Olympic Academy
1750 East Boulder Street
Colorado Springs, CO 80909
(719) 578-4575

United States Olympic Committee
(USOC)
1750 East Boulder Street
Colorado Springs, CO 80909
(719) 632-5551

Physical Education

American Alliance for Health, Physical Education, Recreation and
Dance (AAHPERD)
1900 Association Drive
Reston, VA 22091
(703) 476-3400

National Association for Sport and
  Physical Education
1900 Association Drive
Reston, VA 22091
(703) 476-3410

President's Council on Physical Fitness and Sport
701 Pennsylvania Avenue NW
Suite 250
Washington, DC 20004
(202) 272-3421

Social Sport

North American Society for Sport
  History (NASH)
101 White Building
Penn State University
University Park, PA 16802
(814) 865-2416

North American Society for the
  Psychology of Sport and Physi-
  cal Activity (NASPSPA)
c/o Stephen A. Wallace
University of Colorado, Boulder
Department of Kinesiology
Campus Box 354
Boulder, CO 80307
(303) 492-7333

North American Society for the
  Sociology of Sport (NASSS)
c/o Dr. Howard Nixon
Appalachian State University
Department of Sociology
Boone, NC 28608
(704) 262-2293

Philosophic Society for the Study of
  Sport (PSSS)
c/o Professor Janet M. Oussany
HPER
Kean College of New Jersey
Union, NJ 07083
(201) 527-2101

Sporting Goods

American Society for Testing and
  Materials (ASTM)
1916 Race Street
Philadelphia, PA 19103
(215) 299-5400

Athletic Equipment Managers
  Association
723 Keil Court
Bowling Green, OH 43402
(419) 352-1207

Canadian Sporting Goods Association
1315 de Maisonneuve Boulevard W
Suite 702
Montreal, Quebec, Canada H3G 1M4
(514) 845-6113; Telex 055-61169

National Operating Committee on
  Standards for Athletic Equipment (NOCSE)
11724 Plaza Circle
P.O. Box 202626
Kansas City, MO 64195
(816) 464-5470

National Sporting Goods Association
  (NSGA)
1699 Wall Street
Mount Prospect, IL 60056-5780
(312) 439-4000; Fax (312) 439-4000

Sporting Goods Agents Association
  (SGAA)
P.O. Box 998
Morton Grove, IL 60053
(312) 296-3670

Sporting Goods Manufacturers Association (SGMA)
200 Castlewood Drive
North Palm Beach, FL 33408
(407) 842-4100; Fax (407) 863-8984

Sport Science

Academy for Sports Dentistry
c/o Dr. William Olin
University Hospitals
Iowa City, IA 52242
(319) 356-2601

American Academy of Podiatric
  Sports Medicine (AAPSM)
1729 Glastonberry Road
Potomac, MD 20854
(301) 424-7440

American Academy of Sports
  Physicians (AASP)
17113 Gledhill Street
Northridge, CA 91325
(818) 886-7891

American College of Sports Medicine
P.O. Box 1440
Indianapolis, IN 46206-1440
(317) 637-9200

American Orthopaedic Society for
  Sports Medicine (AOSSM)
2250 East Devon Avenue
Suite 115
Des Plains, IL 60018
(708) 836-7000

American Osteopathic Academy of
  Sports Medicine
7611 Elmwood
Suite 201
Middleton, WI 53562
(608) 831-4400

American Athletic Trainers Association & Certification Board
660 West Duarte Road
Arcadia, CA 91006
(818) 445-1978

Melpomene Institute for Women's
  Health Research
c/o Judy Mahle Lutter
1010 University Avenue
St. Paul, MN 55104
(612) 642-1951

National Strength and Conditioning
  Association
P.O. Box 81410
Lincoln, NE 68501
(402) 472-3000

Women

National Association for Girls and
  Women in Sport
1900 Association Drive
Reston, VA 22091
(703) 476-3450; Fax (703) 476-9527

Women's Sports Foundation
342 Madison Avenue
Suite 72
New York, NY 10173
(212) 972-9170; Fax (212) 949-8024

TRAVEL
AND TOURISM

Air Transport Association
1709 New York Avenue NW
Washington, DC 20006-5206
(202) 626-4000; Fax (202) 626-4181

Airlines Reporting Corporation
1709 New York Avenue NW
Washington, DC 20006
(202) 626-4079

American Automobile Association
8111 Gatehouse Road
Falls Church, VA 22047
(703) 222-6000

American Bus Association
1015 15th Street NW
Suite 250
Washington, DC 20005
(202) 842-1645; Fax (202) 842-0850

American Car Rental Association
2011 Eye Street NW, Fifth Floor
Washington, DC 20006
(202) 223-2118

American Hotel & Motel Association
1201 New York Avenue NW, 6th
  Floor
Washington, DC 20005-3917
(202) 289-3100; Fax (202) 289-3199

American Sightseeing International
309 Fifth Avenue
New York, NY 10016
(212) 689-7744; Fax (212) 686-0818

American Society of Travel Agents
1101 King Street
Alexandria, VA 22314
(703) 739-2782; Fax (703) 684-8319

Arab Tourism Union
POB 2354
Amman, Jordan
Telex 214 71 arabi jo

Association Internationale d'Experts
  Scientifiques du Tourisme
(International Association of Scien-
  tific Experts in Tourism)
Varnbüelstrasse 19
CH-9000
St. Gallen, Switzerland
071 23 55 11

Association of American Railroads
50 F Street NW
Washington, DC 20001
(202) 639-2100; Fax (202) 639-5546

Association of Group Travel
  Executives
c/o The A. H. Light Co., Inc.
424 Madison Avenue
New York, NY 10017
(212) 486-4300

Association of Retail Travel Agents
25 South Riverside
Croton on Hudson, NY 10520
(914) 271-9000; Fax (914) 271-9025

Association of Travel Marketing
  Executives
1776 Massachusetts Avenue NW
#521
Washington, DC 20036
(202) 232-7107

Bureau International du Tourisme
  Social
(International Bureau of Social
  Tourism)
5, Boulevard de l'Imperatrice
B-1000 Brussels, Belgium
2 5140133

Caribbean Tourism Association
20 East 46th Street
New York, NY 10017
(212) 682-0435

Caribbean Tourism Research Centre
Mer Vue, Marine Gardens
Christ Church, Barbados
75242

Council on Hotel, Restaurant and
  Institutional Education
1200 17th Street NW, 7th Floor
Washington, DC 20036-3097
(202) 331-5990; Fax (202) 331-2429

Cruise Lines International Association
500 Fifth Avenue
Suite 1407
New York, NY 10110
(212) 921-0066; Fax (212) 921-0549

East Asia Travel Association
c/o Japan National Tourist Organization
2-10-1 Yurakucho, Chiyoda-Ku
Tokyo, Japan
(03) 216-905

European Travel Commission
2 rue Linois
75015 Paris, France
45.75.62.15; Fax 45.79.90.20

Hotel Sales and Marketing Association International
1300 L Street NW
Suite 800
Washington, DC 20005
(202) 789-0089; Fax (202) 789-1725

Institute of Certified Travel Agents
148 Linden Street
P.O. Box 82-56
Wellesley, MA 02181
(617) 237-0280; (800) 542-4282;
    Fax (617) 237-3860

International Academy of Tourism
9, rue Princesse Marie de Lorraine
Monte Carlo, Monaco
93 309768

International Air Transport Association
2000 Peel Street
Montreal, Quebec, Canada
    PQ H3A 2R4
(514) 844-6311
        &
POB 160, 26 Chemin de Joinville
1216 Cointrin-Geneva, Switzerland
(022) 983366

International Airlines Travel Agent Network
2000 Peel Street
Suite 4060
Montreal, Quebec, Canada
    PQ H3A 2R4
(514) 844-2877; Fax (514) 844-2391

International Association of Amusement Parks and Attractions
4230 King Street
Alexandria, VA 22302
(703) 671-5800; Fax (703) 824-8365

International Association of Conference Centers
900 South Highway Drive
Fenton, MO 63026
(314) 349-5576

International Association of Convention and Visitor Bureaus
P.O. Box 758
Champaign, IL 61824-0758
(217) 359-8881; Fax (217) 359-0965

International Association of Fairs and Expositions
MPO 985
Springfield, MO 65801
(417) 862-5771

International Association of Tour Managers
397 Walworth Road
London, England SE 17 2 AW
01-703-9154; Fax 01-703-0358

International Association of Tour Managers, North American Region
1646 Chapel Street
New Haven, CT 06511
(203) 777-5994

International Civil Aviation Organization
1000 Sherbrooke Street
Montreal, Quebec, Canada
    PQ H3A 2R2
(514) 285-8219

International Congress and Convention Association
P.O. Box 5343
1007 AH
Amsterdam, The Netherlands
020-647421

International Forum of Travel and Tourism Advocates
693 Sutter Street, 6th Floor
San Francisco, CA 94102
(415) 673-3333; Fax (415) 673-3548

Meeting Planners International
Infomart, 1950 Stemmons Freeway
Dallas, TX 75207
(214) 746-5222; Fax (214) 746-5248

National Air Carrier Association
1730 M Street NW
Suite 710
Washington, DC 20036
(202) 833-8200

National Air Transportation
  Association
4226 King Street
Alexandria, VA 22302
(703) 845-9000

National Association of Railroad
  Passengers
236 Massachusetts Avenue NE
Suite 603
Washington, DC 20002
(202) 546-1550

National Business Travel Association
516 Fifth Avenue
Suite 406
New York, NY 10036
(212) 221-6782; Fax (212) 944-5513

National Recreation and Park
  Association
3101 Park Center Drive
Alexandria, VA 22302
(703) 820-4940; Fax (703) 671-4628

National Restaurant Association
1200 17th Street NW
Washington, DC 20036-3097
(202) 331-5900; Fax (202) 331-2429

National Tour Association
P.O. Box 3071
Lexington, KY 40596
(606) 253-1036; Fax (606) 233-1099

Pacific Asia Travel Association
Telesis Tower
1 Montgomery Street
Suite 1750
San Francisco, CA 94104
(415) 986-4646; Fax (415) 986-3458

Pacific Rim Institute of Tourism
P.O. Box 12101
Suite 930-555, West Hastings Street
Vancouver, British Columbia,
  Canada V6B 4N6
(604) 682-8000; Fax (604) 688-2554

Professional Guides Association of
  America
2416 South Eads Street
Arlington, VA 22202
(203) 892-5757

Recreation Vehicle Industry Association
1896 Preston White Drive
Reston, VA 22090
(703) 620-6003; Fax (703) 620-5071

Society for the Advancement of
  Travel for the Handicapped
26 Court Street
Brooklyn, NY 11242
(718) 858-5483; Fax (718) 596-6310

Society of American Travel Writers
1155 Connecticut Avenue NW
Suite 500
Washington, DC 20036
(202) 429-6639

Society of Incentive Travel Executives
271 Madison Avenue
Suite 904
New York, NY 10016-1001
(212) 889-9340; Fax (212) 889-0646

Statistics Canada
International Travel Section
15th Floor, Station J, Coats Building
Ottawa, Ontario, Canada KIA 0T6
(613) 951-8932

&

Travel, Tourism and Recreation
  Section
15A Coats Building
Ottawa, Ontario, Canada KIA 0T6
(613) 951-9169

Tourism Canada
235 Queen Street
Ottawa, Ontario, Canada KIA 0H6
(613) 996-5651

Tourism Industry Association of
  Canada
130 Albert Street
Ottawa, Ontario, Canada KIP 5G4
(613) 238-3883; Fax (613) 238-3878

Travel and Tourism Research Association
P.O. Box 8066, Foothill Station
Salt Lake City, UT 84108
(801) 581-3351

Travel Industry Association of
  America
1133 21st Street NW
Two Lafayette Center
Washington, DC 20036
(202) 293-1433

United States Tour Operators Association
211 East 51st Street
Suite 12B
New York, NY 10022
(212) 944-5727; Fax (202) 421-1285

U.S. Travel Data Center
1133 21st Street NW
Two Lafayette Center
Washington, DC 20036
(202) 293-1040

Universal Federation of Travel
  Agents Associations
Rue Defacqz, 1-Btel
1050 Brussels, Belgium
32-3-5370320; Fax 5374800

World Association for Professional
  Training in Tourism
c/o Españoleto 19-3°
28010 Madrid, Spain

World Association of Travel Agents
37 Quai Wilsons
Geneva, Switzerland 1201
022-731.47.60; Fax 022-732.81.61

World Tourism Organization
Captain Haya 42
28020 Madrid, Spain
5710628; Fax 5713733

AUTHOR/TITLE INDEX

SUBJECT INDEX